OXFORD MEDICAL PU

Therapeutic n. for the
mentally handicapped

Therapeutic nursing
for the
mentally handicapped

ROY D. BAILEY

Senior Clinical Psychologist and
Head of Department of Psychology
The Manor House Hospital,
Aylesbury, Buckinghamshire

OXFORD
OXFORD UNIVERSITY PRESS
NEW YORK TORONTO
1982

Oxford University Press, Walton Street, Oxford OX2 6DP
London Glasgow New York Toronto
Delhi Bombay Calcutta Madras Karachi
Kuala Lumpur Singapore Hong Kong Tokyo
Nairobi Dar es Salaam Cape Town
Melbourne Auckland
and associate companies in
Beirut Berlin Ibadan Mexico City

British Library Cataloguing in Publication Data

Bailey, Roy D.
Therapeutic nursing for the mentally handicapped.
—(Oxford medical publications)
1. Mentally handicapped—Care and treatment
2. Behaviour therapy
I. Title
616.85'880651 RC489.B4

ISBN 0-19-261314-6

Set by The Thetford Press Ltd, Norfolk
Printed in Great Britain by J. W. Arrowsmith Ltd, Bristol

To Anne, Patricia, and Fraser

Contrary to the misconceptions of many, the
retarded do not behave and learn as they do
because of their mental retardation.

William I. Gardener (1972)

Foreword

By
J. BICKNELL

*Professor of the Psychiatry of Mental Handicap
at St. George's Hospital Medical School,
London*

The role of the nurse in the care of the mentally handicapped is changing: in the past the nurse's time was taken up in maintaining the ward routine, protecting those in her charge from all risks, and giving plenty of tender loving care.

Now we expect nursing and other care staff to be as involved in therapeutic procedures as the therapists themselves. The nurse has been asked to change from being an attendant — as indeed nurses were once named — to being a modifier of behaviour, a parent substitute, and an organizer of an exciting life style geared to the needs of the individuals in her charge. Tender loving care has now been enhanced with greater opportunities for teaching daily living skills and testing the limits of realistic independence for all levels of mental handicap.

This book fills a gap in the current nursing literature as it provides a clear account of the theoretical background and practical application of behaviour therapy that the nurse will need if she wishes to become a nurse-therapist and so help those in her care to develop their skills to the full.

Preface

This book is primarily intended for nurses studying and working in the field of mental handicap.* It attempts to provide a systematic framework within which nurses can carry out observation, assessment, therapy planning, and monitoring of therapeutic practice with mentally handicapped children and adolescents. The therapeutic approach outlined is based on psychological principles of observation, assessment, and behaviour therapy. Although not intended to be a 'cookbook' for therapeutic nursing with mentally handicapped people, there is a clear emphasis on how these principles can be applied in practical assessment and therapy. This practical aspect is supported by showing how the nurse can identify therapy targets and teach the mentally handicapped to achieve them — a process which helps the handicapped to reach their full potential.

The text may be used in the education of both nurses in training and qualified nurses who are interested in the psychology of mental handicap. Practical assignments have been included after most chapters so that nurses can gain experience in using the approach to therapy covered in this book. Each assignment should be carried out first by a group and then by each individual nurse. Approaching the assignments in this way allows nurses to build up their skills in therapy gradually. The assignments are intended to test the student's practical and intellectual working knowledge, and become more complex as the book progresses. It should be emphasized that nurses should work in small 'teams' of four to six people. These may include other colleagues, parents, psychologists, social workers, teachers, and, where possible, the mentally handicapped people themselves. The main aim of the assignments is to

* The term 'mental handicap' is used throughout the text to refer to people who are regarded as severely or moderately mentally handicapped. 'Child' is used throughout the book for convenience, although therapy is continued into adolescence and can be begun successfully with adults of any age.

relate training in therapeutic nursing to its *actual* practice. For this reason, wherever possible, real cases rather than simulated problems in mental handicap should be tackled in the assignments.

The assignments are important not only because they test nurses' knowledge but also because they provide them with experience of working individually and in a team. The assignments and exercises undertaken individually or in groups should always be supervised by an appropriately qualified psychologist or tutor. The assignments can then be evaluated by the students and their supervisors, both individually and in group discussion. *In any assignment affecting mentally handicapped children or adolescents the supervisors should ensure there are no medical or ethical reasons why they should not participate in the assignment.*

A training opinion questionnaire has been included for nurses and nurse tutors to use in combination with the personal work assignment sections. Where schools and colleges of nursing are involved, they should be in a position to evaluate the progress of nurse learners' knowledge of the principles and practice of therapeutic nursing with the mentally handicapped. Although primarily written for nurses, this book may also be of theoretical and practical benefit to teachers, social workers, and parents of the mentally handicapped.

Aylesbury   R.D.B.
February 1981

Acknowledgements

It is not easy to remember everyone who in one way or another has provided me with ideas and encouragement to complete this book. I should, however, like to pay special thanks to those of whom I am aware.

Anthony Wilson, Principal Clinical Psychologist, and Andrew Craze, Clinical Psychologist, Department of Psychology, St. Lawrences' Hospital, Bodmin, Cornwall, provided helpful criticism on the earliest formats and the training opinion questionnaire. Alex Prophet, Senior Nursing Officer, Mental Handicap, and Gordon Bath, Nursing Officer, made it possible to carry out the two-year research programme on which some of the current book is based. Dr Alison Tierney, Department of Nursing Studies at the University of Edinburgh, made helpful comments on a later draft and gave me her views on the writing style of the manuscript. In this connection Hazel Allen, Assistant Director of the Kings Fund Centre, has been a major influence in the overall design of the book. I am particularly grateful to her for the idea of including personal work assignments for most of the chapters. Michelle Smith collated and constructed the majority of the material describing some clinical conditions associated with mental handicap. Inclusion of the different assessment scales and reference to others have been possible by the kind permission of Dorothy Jeffree and Roy McConkey, Hester Adrian Research Centre; Nancy Thomson, Principal Clinical Psychologist, Royal Aberdeen Children's Hospital; and the American Association on Mental Deficiency. I am also indebted to Dr Peter Taylor, Dorothy Perkins, and Angus Capie for permission to illustrate the Developmental Checklist devised by them at the British Institute of Mental Handicap. Professor H. C. Gunzburg, Consultant Psychologist, has allowed me to include examples of his Progressive Assessment Charts and contributed two case assessments which are included along with an example courteously supplied by Dr Peter Taylor and Dorothy Perkins. Professor Gunzburg has also given me invaluable intermittent encouragement to complete the manuscript and pointed out some of the finer points of assessment using his PAC Charts. It is also my great pleasure to thank Professor Joan Bicknell, Professor of the Psychiatry of Mental Handicap, for undertaking to read and comment on the final stages of the text. I am also grateful to Dr B. A. Stratford, Consultant Psychiatrist in Mental Handicap, for contributing Appendix 2 on drug use in mental handicap. My appreciation is extended to the Oxford University Press who demonstrated a sustained interest in the manuscript and offered helpful editorial advice.

Melita Smith and Maureen Marriott wrestled with my handwriting to produce the final typewritten draft. To them I express my sincere thanks for completing a task which could only have added to their already busy work schedule.

Contents

1

The idea of therapeutic nursing

THERAPY

Traditionally much of the therapy that nurses working with the mentally handicapped have been involved in can be broadly classified as 'medical'. In this sense therapy has been aimed at treating an illness or a disease. The idea of therapeutic nursing outlined in this book is concerned with therapy of a different kind. This kind of therapy is composed of systematic courses of assessment and actions which can be carried out by nurses to help mentally handicapped children and adolescents develop through learning. The learning which each mentally handicapped child has acquired can be seen in the range of behaviour which he exhibits at home, school, hospital, and with family and friends. Some behaviour displayed by the mentally handicapped tends to be described in terms which are difficult to assess and this makes it hard to employ therapy which can be observed and monitored. When this happens therapeutic nursing may be 'successful', but it may be difficult to identify at which points the successes took place. When therapy fails, this may be due to a variety of factors. The mentally handicapped person's problems may have been incorrectly diagnosed, or perhaps the diagnosis was correct but the therapy plan was inappropriate. In this sort of situation it is not surprising that nurses' efforts at therapy often do not produce clear results. To resolve these issues it is necessary to provide a conceptionalization of therapy which helps to identify the targets for therapy; the way in which therapy is to proceed; how it is to be monitored; and how it is to be evaluated. A behavioural approach to helping the mentally handicapped fulfils these requirements, and involves the sort of therapy which can be carried out by nurses. 'Behaviour therapy' is the application of systems of rewards and penalties which maintain, increase, or decrease a person's behaviour.

The behavioural approach to therapeutic nursing, however, should not ignore the basic emotional and educational needs of the mentally handicapped. Although there is a wide range of disabilities shown by mentally handicapped children (see Appendix 1) it should be remembered their *needs* are broadly the same as the so-called 'normal population'. The behavioural approach to therapy should be used to promote fulfilment of these needs — alongside the development of self-help skills such as toiletting, feeding, dressing, communication, play, personal independence, and the formation of friendships. Before beginning this therapeutic nursing it is imperative to recognize and accept that every handicapped child is first a person in their own right, and only secondly a handicapped person. Identifying psychological needs should be a primary consideration when assessing the mentally handicapped as this reflects the ethics of therapy as well as the kind of therapy to be carried out.

PSYCHOLOGICAL NEEDS OF THE MENTALLY HANDICAPPED

It is not possible to list all of the mentally handicapped child's needs but there are a number which deserve close consideration when assessing children who may be considered for therapy. The first of these is *the need to give and receive affection*. All mentally handicapped children need to give love and to be liked and loved for themselves — not for the kinds of 'tricks' that they might be able to perform for their parents, teachers, social workers, nursing personnel, or other 'normal' people. A bond of affection between the caregiver and the child is often necessary before any valid assessment or therapy can begin. This affection should not be conditional in the first instance, but should be aimed at simply satisfying the emotional needs of the child. Whoever occupies the role of the behaviour therapist should communicate their recognition of these needs. It is the right of each mentally handicapped child to expect such recognition.* The same can be said of the mentally handicapped child's *need to feel secure*. In behavioural terms this can be interpreted as having a family who are consistent and stable. If this is not possible, then it is important to have a family substitute to satisfy the need for security. Hospitals, adoptive families, foster parents, and hostels should

* Declaration of Human Rights United Nations (1971).

strive to provide protection and friendship in a place like home if children are unable to stay with their own parents or other family (HMSO 1971). A familiar place to work and play; to be with people they know who behave in a predictable way, and who set guidelines for their conduct will help to fulfil their basic psychological need for security. Nurses should recognize this as an important need which must be met before therapy can begin.

However, it is not enough that mentally handicapped children should feel secure and receive tender loving care (Bailey and Patterson 1977). They also need to be *recognized and accepted as individuals who achieve goals by their own efforts*. This is one of the most important points to remember when drawing up any therapy plan aimed at promoting personal development in the mentally handicapped. All children need to be valued and recognized for their own efforts when they are trying to learn and achieve things. Recognition and appropriate reward for their efforts should communicate to them a feeling of self-satisfaction. This contributes to their well-being. The psychological term used to describe this sense of well-being, is 'self-esteem'. Like normal children mentally handicapped children can have low, moderate, or high self-esteem. When the level of self-esteem is judged by a person's behaviour it is possible to measure it and to record how often the child shows various levels of self-esteem. The task for the nurse should be to assist the child to achieve a high level of self-esteem. In looser terms, nurses should help children to accept themselves. So if, for example, therapy were aimed at trying to promote brushing shoes or clean eating habits, the child would be recognized and rewarded for his achievement. This should in turn increase his self-esteem. It is not necessary or always desirable to promote competitiveness amongst mentally handicapped children. In the first instance, they may differ in their individual abilities to learn to compete for any set therapeutic goal, but secondly, and equally important, since mentally handicapped children need to be valued for themselves, it is imprudent to compare them with each other in this way. Therapeutic nursing should not aim at competitiveness. But it is of great importance for mentally handicapped children that they are recognized for trying their best. One child's effort may produce poor results than another's, but the effort he has put into, say, imitating speech or doing up a zip, may be greater. A helpful rule-of-thumb to employ in therapeutic nursing is to direct therapy at the level where the child can succeed, then move on to more difficult tasks and goals. Start and end with success. This is of primary significance for a great deal of work with mentally handicapped children. They may easily already regard themselves as failures. If therapy is to be successful in any way, it should not start or end with failure. Like normal children, the mentally handicapped are not motivated by failure; they are motivated to learn as a result of previous success in learning.

Each mentally handicapped child should also be given the opportunity of learning through their own experience of the world. This means that *mentally handicapped children have the need to repeat known experiences and learn through expanding what they have already learnt into new experiences*. This is usually best achieved by varying the experiences of each child within a set therapeutic and developmental structure. In this way it is also possible to provide each child with new experiences which are learnt. In other words it should be part of the nurse's therapeutic effort to provide a variety of experiences within each child's range of abilities. These should be gradually expanded to include new learning from new experiences.

Unlike normal children most mentally handicapped children do not usually initiate their own experiences in learning to dress, walk-explore, play, or talk. This is obviously due to various degrees of neurological damage resulting in various degrees of mental handicap. From the point of view of learning and behaviour therapy, it also means such children do not have the abilities of normal children to learn from ambiguous learning situations. Normal children actively learn through their experience of the world and also begin very early to structure their own learning. In addition to structuring their own learning, normal children transfer what they have learnt from one situation to another. So normal children also employ economy of learning. Another characteristic of normal learning is the way in which children experiment with what they have learnt in order to gain deeper understanding from their experience of their world and the effect they have on it. Mentally handicapped children are often without these abilities to learn and structure learning, or experiment with what they have learnt. As a result, the vital learning through movement, play, and language which occurs for the normal child, often has to be clearly and systematically taught to the mentally handicapped child. This is one of the main aims of therapeutic nursing. The nurse as behaviour therapist should be concerned with teaching mentally handicapped children *how* to learn as well as *what* to learn. Where there are physical handicaps in addition to mental handicap, children are often prevented from actively exploring their surroundings. If left disregarded, the barriers imposed by physical handicap curtail exploration and the growth of personal independence. Providing there is no medical reason why movement should not be encouraged, vigorous therapeutic effort should be made to help children to explore and investigate their surroundings through the movements of their own bodies. Encouraging movement, even in the most severe cases, gives a minimal level of independence and personal control.

The need for some measure of independence and social competence is sometimes overlooked when considering therapy with mentally handicapped children. Our larger institutions, in particular the traditional mental hospitals, have not made enough constructive efforts to promote the need for personal independence. However, it is fair to say that greater efforts have been made recently to help the mentally handicapped achieve various levels of social competence. It is important not to confuse social competence with conformity to behaviour expected by a large institution like the hospital or special school. Each child needs to develop an idea of who he or she is as an individual. Misinformed thinking and planning of mental handicap services can deprive the mentally handicapped of experiencing some level of independence and personal control over their environment on the ill-founded grounds that it is 'beyond their capabilities'. These judgements should not be made without giving the mentally handicapped an opportunity to learn from doing more for themselves and rewarding them for their efforts. Since many of the mentally handicapped spend a great deal of their time in a limited range of settings, hospital, home, hostel, training centre and school, it is of great importance whom they live with, and under what sorts of living conditions. A considerable degree of *choice* should also be offered to the mentally handicapped, especially in their choice of friends, clothing, personal possessions, and living accommodation. Where this is possible, a greater measure of personal independence should result and a truer level of social competence. As mentally handicapped children learn to achieve a greater degree of personal independence and social competence, they will be in a better position to fulfil *their need for friendship and acceptance by other people,* both handicapped and normal alike. However, mentally handicapped children often have to be guided in their interactions with others. This means that practising therapy will often have to address itself to 'priming' interactions between mentally handicapped children and adults. Making friends, and being accepted, depends a great deal on appropriate social behaviour (Trower, Bryant, and Argyle 1978). The most obvious example of achieving these behaviours is encouraging and rewarding the child for sharing in a group. Whether in hospital, school, or at home, it is the responsibility of normal peers and adults to teach the child when to share, and when sharing is *not* appropriate.

All of these psychological needs of the mentally handicapped are also the needs of normal children. Mentally handicapped children often take longer to acquire ways of fulfilling their needs. In some cases these may never be fulfilled or are only achieved after many years of learning. An important task for therapeutic nursing is to organize learning experiences for mentally handicapped children so that their needs can be realized. The first step in behaviour therapy is to recognize and identify these needs. From this point, being guided by what is known about normal development in children helps to provide the sorts of goals therapy should aspire to achieve. When this has been done, the essential belief that all mentally handicapped children can learn to various degrees can be put into organized therapeutic nursing practice.

The development of each child can be promoted by parents, nurses, teachers, and social workers, employing systems of assessment, observation, therapy planning, therapy practice, and therapy evaluation.

2

Therapeutic strategies

BASIC BELIEFS

Good tender loving care is very important for mentally handicapped children, but it is not enough to fulfil their psychological needs and promote their personal development (Bailey and Patterson 1977). Nurses should aim to develop therapeutic strategies. This short chapter attempts to illustrate fundamental stages by which this might be achieved.

Every time a person interacts with a handicapped child, there is an opportunity for therapy. The nurse can act as therapist and help the child to learn something new, or maintain and establish learning which has already been achieved. Nurses should be able to do this in their daily practice. 'Natural' opportunities for therapeutic nursing do occur — for instance, in dressing, feeding, toiletting, and communication. Any therapeutic strategies which nurses adopt should aim to make learning structured and enjoyable for each individual. The main aims of therapeutic strategies are to promote the development of self-help skills, communication, independence, and socially acceptable behaviour. The outcome of these efforts has practical benefits for both the nurses and the children. Nurses who use therapeutic strategies experience an increase in their morale and job satisfaction. The children advance their personal development.

One point must be clear in the minds of 'old' and 'new' nursing personnel, teachers, and social workers officially employed in the field of mental handicap. Most mentally handicapped children do not 'pick things up' with the ease that their normal peers do. They do not have a driving curiosity to explore constructively and to understand readily the world they live in and the demands made of them by society. However, mentally handicapped children can learn and do respond well to planned therapy. Planning therapy must come from providing each child with an individual assessment of their development and psychological needs. Just as we all learn what behaviour is expected of us in different situations, the mentally handicapped child has the right to be shown clearly what behaviour the nurse as behaviour therapist expects him to learn. Additionally, the nurse should adopt therapeutic strategies which show the child how to achieve different kinds of skills and behaviour. Similarly the nurse also needs clear and systematic guidance on the best way to formulate and carry out therapeutic strategies. This means tailor-making therapy for the child and not fitting the children to what happens to be convenient for the personnel or for the routine of the home, hospital, or school they attend. This issue will also be raised again when we discuss problem behaviour and the practice of therapeutic nursing.

There are no two children alike in all respects, whether they are normal or mentally handicapped. Because of this, it is essential to have an individual investigation plan for constructing therapeutic strategies. When the plan has been carried out the nurse should then be in a position to begin therapy. This approach is also vital for deciding which therapeutic strategy to adopt in order to encourage personal development and desirable behaviour.

DESIGNING A THERAPEUTIC STRATEGY

Designing an effective therapeutic strategy to help promote the child's development should consist of at least five connected phases. The first phase of a therapeutic strategy is *assessment*. If an assessment is systematically conducted it will provide the basis for the rest of the therapeutic strategy. The second phase is closely connected with assessment, and is called the *observation and recording* phase. Planning therapeutic strategies for nursing will often mean observing and recording *what* each child can do, *where* they do it, *how it is done, when* and *how often*. Nurses engaged in producing therapy plans should be able to present a detailed personal assessment profile of each individual child's behaviour. Doing this allows them to make careful and accurate decisions about what therapy to employ, e.g. the type of therapy techniques that should be adopted to reduce problem behaviours such as kicking, biting, and punching. This also applies to other areas of development, such as self-care skills and social competence. When the assessment and observation phases are completed, therapy targets or goals can then be set by the nurse. After this the *formulation* phase should be designed. This entails the formulation of a therapeutic strategy which can be put into observable practice. The practice of therapeutic strategy is often referred to as the *action* phase of therapy. Any therapeutic strategy which cannot be practised and seen *in* practice is bad therapeutic nursing. The action phase of therapy should also permit it to be monitored any time during the life of the therapy plan. This means that there is also a *continuous evaluation* phase which should be continuously monitored to established the effectiveness of the therapeutic strategy. Such an approach also fulfils the important function of informing the nurse at any one time the effect therapy may be having on a child's behaviour.

Planning therapy is a crucial component of therapeutic strategies and absolutely essential in estimating later therapeutic effects of any therapy plan. In the first instance, planning therapy and implementing a therapeutic strategy should be supervised by a suitably qualified clinical psychologist who specializes in mental handicap. Ideally, and in practice, a working dialogue between members of the therapeutic team should be encouraged with the explicit aim of discovering and providing a practical framework to achieve realistic behavioural and developmental goals for each child. In many ways this means that the team must work within clearly stated procedures laid down in the therapeutic strategy, and in concordance with each of its different phases. The basic therapeutic strategy can be helpfully summarized under five main categories:

(1) assessment;
(2) observation;
(3) therapy formulation;
(4) therapeutic practice — action phase;
(5) continuous assessment — evaluation.

It is the organized and co-ordinated practice of all these components which constitutes the therapeutic strategy and characterizes therapeutic nursing.

Each stage of the therapeutic strategy should be completed before moving on to the next. Assessment should be designed to provide information along with observations which suggest the therapy to be practised. The continuous assessment of the therapy being practised should also be recorded in such a way that it makes sense to anyone involved. In this way a wealth of relevant information can be intelligibly shared between nursing colleagues, psychologists, social workers, teachers, parents, and where possible the handicapped children themselves.

3

Assessment

RELEVANCE AND PRACTICAL VALUE

There are a number of questions asked about the psychological assessment of the mentally handicapped. One of the most frequent is — 'Why is it important to assess mentally handicapped children?' There is no short answer that satisfies every aspect of this question, but from a psychological point of view, assessment should be carried out with the intention of helping individuals develop and fulfil their needs so far as their learning will permit. This will often mean that therapy should be aimed at promoting learning. 'Programme' is the common shorthand term used to refer to various sorts of therapy plans. It is important that mentally handicapped children should have these programmes fitted to them rather than their being fitted to therapy generally available. This is a principle which applies to every mentally handicapped child and is one that can be overlooked in the day-to-day events affecting their lives. In order to achieve person-fitted behaviour therapy, we must have a clear idea of what each individual can do, or cannot do or does not currently do already.

In assessing a mentally handicapped child it is important to have a personal profile of his strengths and weaknesses with regard to any particular skill and learning. When this has been done, we are in a better position to devise an effective nursing therapy plan. The plan should be designed to provide practical and realistic ways of building on his strengths whilst attempting to ameliorate his weaknesses. The nurse should ideally aim to change the child's behaviour so that he can live a fuller and more independent life. Assessment is the key to planning the therapy which will help to realize these goals.

The assessment phase of therapy is often ignored when trying to help the mentally handicapped to develop their skills and learning. It should be emphasized that assessment is crucial to successful therapeutic practice. A disciplined attitude and practice can be usefully cultivated in at least four areas of assessment. These are briefly outlined in the personal assessment profile shown below.

TABLE 3.1

Personal assessment profile

Area	Questions
1. *General assessment*	Has the child a mental handicap? Has the child an emotional handicap? Has the child a physical handicap? Has the child some form of multiple handicap? Are there any typical syndromes and effects displayed by the handicapping condition?
2. *Specific assessment*	What range of handicaps does this child have? How severe are they? How does his level of performance compare with other mentally handicapped children? How does his level of performance compare with normal people of his age group? What is his rate of learning for different skills and other behaviour? What style of therapy-teaching does he respond to best?
3. *Therapy plan assessment*	What do the general and specific areas of assessment tell us about planning therapy? How and in what way should therapy progress? What behaviours should be part of the therapeutic practice to help the handicapped child achieve new behaviours and develop his skills through learning?
4. *Therapy practice assessment*	What behaviours are to count as indicators of successful therapeutic practice? How long should it be before they occur? Who is to practise the therapy plan? How are the effects of therapeutic practice to be monitored, recorded, and evaluated?

All these points should be closely considered in the earliest phases of therapy. This means developing a systematic approach to the assessment of each child. Gone are the days of 'on-the-spot' diagnosis. The most helpful assessment that can be made for the mentally handicapped is to assess their need for therapy which promotes learning new and desirable behaviours. The mentally handicapped are not primarily ill and are not, therefore, a medical problem. This does not mean to say that drugs and medication are not helpful. However, it is fair to say that many such drugs do not promote learning. In many instances they actually impair the already limited learning ability of the mentally handicapped, for example some anti-epileptic drugs have toxic side-effects, and certain combinations of drugs can lead to impaired functioning (see Appendix 2).

For the practical purposes of therapeutic nursing, nurses should always aim to define a clear therapy plan and decide how they are going to put it into practice and evaluate it. When this has been decided, they should be consistent and practise therapy in the way it has been planned. The golden rule of therapeutic nursing therefore is to practise the therapy plan in the job. Therapy is never therapy until it is practised.

THE TOOLS OF ASSESSMENT

There are many types of assessment used by clinical psychologists to assess the mentally handicapped. Developmental scales and developmental checklists are used a great deal. These are tests designed to assess various behaviours in a person's development and are often useful in planning therapy. Although not ideal, they provide a constructive and systematic starting-point for assessing the handicapped child. But developmental scales and developmental checklists should not be treated as an end in themselves. With this in mind, it is often wise to consult colleagues and other professionals such as psychologists when therapy plans are being formulated. The following developmental scales are useful in assessing a mentally handicapped child. Selecting an appropriate scale should depend on the degree of the person's mental handicap and the range of behaviour to be assessed.

1. **The Adaptive Behaviour Scale for Children and Adults.** This is an American scale for assessing behaviour across a wide range of development. It is basically a checklist, but it also introduces the therapist to assessing the *frequency* of behaviours recorded.

2. **The Parental Involvement Project developmental charts.** The PIP charts were developed after a survey of the characteristics of normal children had been made and the results incorporated into the final scales. The charts are often used by parents and other caregivers to estimate the level of development and functioning

level of each child. The charts also serve to introduce all caregivers to the idea and importance of objective measurement. Therapy targets can be selected from the PIP charts, but this is usually done by further detailed observation and investigation of possible therapy targets.

3. **The Gunzburg Progress Assessment Charts.** These are actually a comprehensive range of different 'social competence' charts. Commonly referred to as 'the PAC' they are perhaps the most well-known scales and can be used with children, adolescents, and adults with various levels of mental handicap. The scales are regularly reviewed by Professor Gunzburg (the innovator of the PACs). From time to time amendments are made to the charts to improve the quality of the scales. Consulting the various manuals which are guides to scoring and calculating a mentally handicapped person's social competence profile is an essential requirement when using the PAC. Some of the scales also permit caregivers to make a general assessment of the 'personality' of the mentally handicapped person. However, this is a more subjective assessment than the social competence part of the PACs.

4. **The Developmental Checklist.** This checklist was developed at The British Institute of Mental Handicap (formerly the Institute of Mental Subnormality). It is based on general child development in the first five years of life. The areas of development are divided up into different sections of development for the convenience of systematic assessment. A helpful and clear scoring system is provided for the assessor. Another useful aspect of this checklist is that it also shows what therapy targets the mentally handicapped person should learn *next* in his personal development. It can therefore be employed both as an assessment tool and as an aid for identifying individual targets which can be used to plan therapy.

5. **The Raeden Development Assessment Guide.** This developmental guide was constructed from a combination of other developmental scales. Emphasis in using this guide is on the individual and his developmental profile over time and in different situations. Although the guide shows estimated levels of child development in months on the scale, this is only supposed to be used as a general comparative guideline. The Raeden guide is best used when the child or adolescent is compared with his *own* progress and his *own* development. Using the Raeden scales it is primarily the development of each individual child within himself, rather than comparison with others which should concern the nurse.

All of these developmental scales are in use in the United Kingdom. Further details of the scales and addresses where they can be obtained are given in the list on p.144. However, it may help to illustrate how some of the scales have been used. In order to do this three examples are included here showing sections of selected scales and the way the assessment was reported.

THE PROGRESS ASSESSMENT CHART FORM 1 (PAC1)

Case 1

The PAC Form 1 was used to assess 'Charles'. The assessor carried out a social and personal development assessment. Working through each section of the scale, areas Charles passed were shaded in on the PAC assessment discs. Where he had no opportunity to learn specified skills 'NO' was entered against the item and on the social assessment diagram. Where the assessment was 'not appropriate' 'NA' was marked against items and chart. Areas still to be learnt may be left blank or a line drawn through each box. The areas of development where the lines have been drawn through represent gaps in Charles's development. The PAC shows Charles's current levels of social and personal development (see Fig 3.1).

Social assessment

Compared with other 16-year-old mentally handicapped children living in the open community, Charles must certainly be regarded as 'backward' in the three main areas of self-help (76 per cent); communication (85 per cent); and occupation (85 per cent). Only in the area of socialization is his overall attainment average (100 per cent).

The PAC record suggests that Charles's backwardness is not necessarily due only to his mental handicap or even his muteness. There are 13 NOs marked in the record, which indicate that the institutional regime deprives him of a substantial slice of important life experience. It is absolutely essential for Charles's development (and that of others) to change these faulty management practices, particularly since they are not necessary to the running of the institution. There is also very suggestive evidence that Charles is much brighter than either his IQ or the general level of achievement suggest. His attainments in the subsections of 'number work' and 'paper and pencil work' are very good and it can be assumed with some confidence that a planned programme for developing comprehension of the spoken

Fig. 3.1.

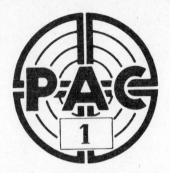

PROGRESS ASSESSMENT CHART
OF SOCIAL AND PERSONAL DEVELOPMENT
(For the Mentally Handicapped)

FORM 1
12th Edition
by
H. C. GUNZBURG, M.A., Ph.D., F.B.Ps.S.

Oak House

(Name of Teaching Centre)

Name   Charles Jones   Sex M   Date of Birth 5.8.65   Age 16+

Address

Date of Assessment 10.9.81   Signature of Assessor   *MB*

EXAMPLE:

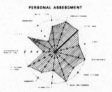

This 14-year old boy has obtained a good average score in the SELF-HELP section of the P-A-C 1, and is very good in the COMMUNICA TION section compared with other mentally handicapped children of his age. He is functioning well in the SOCIALISATION and OCCUPATION areas, though he should certainly be encouraged to help around the house. On the whole, this boy functions well considering his age and mental level, but the "filling-in" of some noticeable gaps would make him into a "better than average" m.h. boy. His personal assessment diagram shows that he is generally very acceptable and, probably, a very likeable boy despite his short-lived temper outbursts. He still needs checking of personal appearance and personal hygiene, but these particular shortcomings in a boy of his age are of comparatively little importance considering his general functioning.

BEFORE marking the diagrams, READ the instructions on the back page of this form.

The criteria for assessment are found in the P - A - C Manual, 3rd edition.

PERSONAL ASSESSMENT

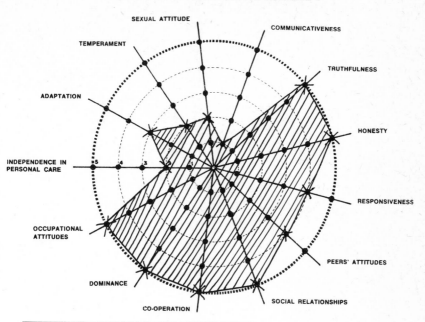

Any physical defect?—describe Mutism	Has to be given medication.................... Could be/is responsible for own medication............ No medication given....................✔	Conspicuous (C) or 'Normal' (N) appearance? N

INDEPENDENCE IN PERSONAL CARE
1. Needs maximum attention . . . .
✔ 2. Needs a helping hand and/or constant checking . . . .
3. A final checking by others is necessary . . . .
4. Quite acceptable standards . . . .
5. Quite superior level of attainment compared with his peers . . . .

ADAPTATION
1. Psychotic behaviour, unconcerned with the world around him . . . .
2. Eccentric—hyperactive—obsessive behaviour . . . .
✔ 3. Hypochondriacal—paranoid tendencies . . . .
4. Inadequate—shortsighted—bad tempered . . . .
5. No 'abnormal' socially disturbing behaviour . . . .

TEMPERAMENT
1. Temper outbursts (screams, yelling, etc.) . . . .
✔ 2. Irritable, short-lived flare-ups, etc. . . . .
3. Swings of mood which are more of a nuisance than up-setting . . . .
4. On the whole even tempered, and if upset equilibrium is restored fairly quickly . . . .
5. Always or nearly always even tempered . . . .

SEXUAL ATTITUDE
1. Severe unacceptable sexual behaviour, e.g., exposure, rape . . . .
✔ 2. Disturbing sexual behaviour, e.g., homosexuality, pro-miscuousness . . . .
3. Behaviour reflects need for affection and may interfere with adjustment . . . .
4. On the whole no interest in particular relationships . . . .
5. Has friendships with people of opposite sex . . . .

COMMUNICATIVENESS
✘ 1. Scarcely any interest in communication—though he may chatter to himself . . . .
2. Repetitive—inconsistent—irrelevant—inaccurate and one-sided communication . . . .
3. Replies to questions and volunteers information occa-sionally . . . .
4. Communication limited to a few interests which are 'discussed' rather than forced on the listener . . . .
5. A good informant on most topics relating to own life . . . .

TRUTHFULNESS
1. Frequently tells deliberate lies, spontaneously and mis-chievously . . . .
2. Tells lies to avoid rebuke—embroiders or exaggerates—tells attention-seeking lies . . . .
3. Accounts given are not always truthful and reliable since he occasionally gets confused . . . .
4. Most of the time he can be believed but will be evasive to avoid trouble . . . .
✔ 5. Can be relied on to speak the truth even though he may not volunteer it . . . .

HONESTY
1. Is light-fingered or quite unscrupulous in his transac-tions . . . .
2. Pilfers occasionally . . . .
3. Helps himself—borrows without permission—may forget to return other people's property . . . .
4. Honest, but accepts advantages when they come his way . . . .
✔ 5. Thoroughly honest and respects other people's property . . . .

RESPONSIVENESS
1. Sulks—frequent ups and downs—rude ....
2. Easily misled—exploited by others ....
3. Keeps himself to himself but is accessible ....
4. Is fairly responsive but attaches himself to only a few people .... ✓
5. Is at ease with most people and responds readily ...

PEERS' ATTITUDES
1. Generally speaking, he is disliked and rejected by most ....
2. Others take little or no notice of him most of the time ....
3. Tolerated by others—has a few 'friends' ....
4. Generally speaking, quite popular and better liked than most .... ✗
5. Other people take their 'cue' from him and follow his example ....

SOCIAL RELATIONSHIPS
1. Solitary—lives generally in a world of his own ....
2. Is demonstrative—interfering—attention-seeking ....
3. Does not look for personal relationships even though he may want them ....
4. Relates well with one or two people .... ✓
5. Relationships with most people are very good ....

CO-OPERATION
1. Refuses frequently to co-operate—usually passive—verbally or physically aggressive ....
2. Co-operation usually short-lived—not very responsive—poor concentration ....
3. As a rule co-operates willingly ....
4. Offers sometimes extra help and assistance .... ✓
5. Wishes to please people and is most willing ...

DOMINANCE
1. Frequently physically aggressive ....
2. Likes to throw his weight about, bosses other people, causes squabbles ....
3. One of a crowd, accepts orders ....
4. Stands up for himself when there is need ... ✓
5. Accepts the rights of others who are in a weaker position ....

OCCUPATIONAL ATTITUDES
1. Restless and unsettled ....
2. Over-entnusiasm interferes with people and occupation ....
3. Fairly settled and carries on with occupation mechanically ....
4. Asks for guidance and responds to it ....
5. Shows some measure of 'initiative' .... ✓

The P-A-C and P-E-I

PURPOSE: The P-A-C provides a visual check of functioning and progress in the four main areas of social development and in various aspects of personal development. Statements referring to relevant skills and behaviour are listed in the inventories of the P-A-C and achievements and deficiencies are thus pinpointed with some accuracy. The diagrams provide not only visual records of present functioning but relate successes and failures to efficiency levels and degrees of social acceptability. They should be compared with the diagrams of previous assessments. Re-assessments indicate whether remedial education and training have been effective.

THE SOCIAL ASSESSMENT: Shade heavily all areas in the diagram where the trainee is competent. **Shade lightly** areas, where the necessary competence has not been acquired yet. **Leave blank** all those areas which cannot be adequately assessed for one or the other reason. Make re-assessments at regular six-monthly intervals.

The Social Competence Index (SCI) indicates clearly the trainee's level of functioning in each of the four areas, compared with his peers ((see P-A-C Manual, 3rd Edition, pp. 137-143).

The Progress Evaluation Index (P-E-I) gives an opportunity for comparing a trainee's progress visually with his peers in course of a number of re-assessments.

THE PERSONAL ASSESSMENT: This rating procedure relates various aspects of personal functioning to degrees of acceptability in the open community. Each radius, referring to a particular aspect, contains a 5-point scale with the highest point (5) indicating the most acceptable behaviour which can reasonably be required from a mentally handicapped person, whilst the lowest point (1) refers to the most unacceptable level of behaviour. Mark one point on each radius and connect the points on the various radii with lines. Shade in the area within the connecting lines to obtain an irregularly shaped figure. Generally speaking, the larger the area, the better the level of social acceptability; the smaller the area, the greater the adjustment difficulties.

When the two diagrams of the P-A-C are studied side by side, it will be possible to judge how far 'good' social attainments on the social diagram are supported by 'good' personal ratings in the personal diagram (indicated by the shaded area extending mostly to points 4 and 5). If a 'good' social diagram is accompanied by a 'meagre' personal diagram (shaded area mostly below points 3), it can readily be appreciated that such a person will not easily be integrated into the open community despite good social competence (see P-A-C Manual, 3rd Edition, pp. 145-156).

GENERAL REMARKS. The **P-A-C 1** is particularly useful for the age groups 6-16 years. If the child is a 'mongol' (Down's syndrome) the **M/P-A-C 1** should be used for assessment. Children who score fairly well on the **P-A-C 1** should also be assessed on the green **P-A-C 1A** which contains a wider range of social skills within the competence of the senior child. Very young or profoundly mentally handicapped children should be assessed on the **P**(rimary)-**P-A-C**. Note that P-A-C forms should be used as appropriate to the level of functioning—and age should not be regarded as the decisive factor (see P-A-C Manual). The **P-A-C 2** has been designed for teenagers and older mentally handicapped people.

The assessment on this chart represents the first vital step towards an individualised programme which is based on the diagnosis of specific weaknesses. Since the P-A-C identifies underdeveloped abilities in need of special attention, the assessment provides also an itemised teaching programme for further action.

It will be necessary to establish whether a particular child is 'average,' 'superior' or 'backward' in social attainments **compared with mentally handicapped children of the same age.** The Progress Evaluation Index (P-E-I) has been developed to give opportunities for comparing the achievements of a particular child, assessed on the P-A-C, with the 'average attainments' in the various subsections of the P-A-C, as achieved by different age groups of mentally handicapped children. The results of a **P-A-C 1** record should be recorded on the **P-E-I 1**, the **P-P-A-C** on the **P-P-E-I,** and the **P-A-C 2** on the **P-E-I 2.** Mongol children, who have been assessed on the **M/P-A-C 1,** should have their achievements entered in the **M/P-E-I 1.** (There is a 'male' and 'female' **M/P-E-I** available, because the 'average achievements' vary according to the sex of the child and care should be taken in selecting the correct P-E-I folder.)

> USE at all times the P-A-C Manual (3rd Edition) for scoring criteria and interpretation

Name... Charles Jones .... Age .16 years, 1 month

SOCIAL ASSESSMENT

SCI(SH)

76%

SCI(C)

85%

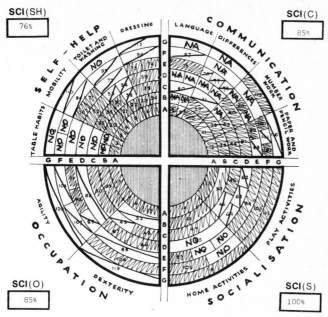

SCI(O)

85%

SCI(S)

100%

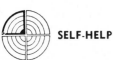

SELF-HELP

Table Habits

✓	1.	Uses spoon when eating without requiring help	A
✓	2.	Drinks without spilling, holding glass in one hand	A
NO	18.	Uses fork without difficulty (food may be cut and prepared)	B
NO	19.	Capable of helping himself to a drink	B
O	34.	Serves himself and eats without requiring much help	C
O	51.	Uses table knife for spreading butter, jam, etc.	D
O	69.	Uses table knife for cutting without much difficulty	E
O	92.	Uses knife and fork correctly and without difficulty	F
O	93.	Pours liquids (e.g., coffee, milk)	F
O	109.	Uses knife for peeling fruit or slicing bread	G

Only 2 items have been credited, though one would expect 8 'successes' at this age. This considerable backwardness might be due to 'NO' - the youth having been brought up to eat his ration of food only with a spoon. No opportunities have been provided for helping oneself to food and drink. There is a great need for normalized environmental conditions.

Mobility

✓	3.	Walks upstairs, both feet together on each step	A
✓	4.	Walks downstairs, both feet together on each step	A
✓	20.	Uses play vehicle of some kind	B
✓	35.	Walks upstairs, one foot per step, without supporting himself	C
✓	36.	Walks downstairs, one foot per step, without supporting himself	C
✓	52.	Goes to neighbours and places nearby	D
✓	70.	Requires little supervision playing outside house, absent for one hour or more	E
✓	71.	Roams about without need for much supervision	E
–	94.	Goes about neighbourhood unsupervised, but does not cross streets	F
–	110.	Goes about neighbourhood unsupervised, crosses streets	G

Eight items have been credited although only 5 skills are expected at this level. This superior achievement may be the result of a generally very relaxed discipline and little supervision, but whatever the reason, Charles's behaviour does not seem to cause concern. Charles may well be ready to be taught the skills required in crossing streets.

Toilet and Washing

✓	5. "Toilet-trained" with infrequent "accidents"	A
✓	21. Asks to go to the toilet or goes by himself	B
✓	22. Dries hands adequately without much assistance	B
✓	37. Cares for himself at the toilet and cleans himself	C
—	38. Washes his hands with soap in an acceptable way	C
—	53. Washes face more or less adequately (not necessarily behind ears)	D
—	54. Brushes his teeth	D
—	72. Tidies hair at regular intervals	E
—	95. Washes himself adequately and completely without much supervision	F
NO	111. Prepares everything for washing himself (e.g., runs bath and assembles what is needed, soap, towel)	G

Only 4 out of the expected 8 skills at this age! - a poor show. All the 'washing skills' seem to be inadequate for this age and it will be necessary to place far more emphasis on this aspect in future.

Dressing

✓	6. Pulls off socks	A
✓	7. Assists in getting dressed	A
✓	23. Removes **and** puts on simple articles of clothing	B
✓	24. Unbuttons accessible buttons	B
✓	39. Fastens and adjusts his clothing	C
✓	55. Undresses at night with little supervision	D
✓	73. Dresses in the morning with little supervision	E
✓	74. Puts on most ordinary articles of clothing	E
	96. Ties shoelaces	F
—	112. Ties a tie (boys), ties a bow, e.g., hair ribbon or apron (girls)	G

Eight out of 10, an average achievement for his age group. The 2 missing skills are not likely to be learnt soon because the institution administration favours slip-on shoes and neither ties nor ribbons are in general use.

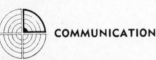 **COMMUNICATION**

Language

✓	8. Obeys simple instructions	A
—	9. **Understands** orders containing: on, in, behind, under, above, in front of, on top, underneath	A
NA	25. Relates experiences in a coherent way	B
NA	26. Sentences contain plurals, past tense, "I," prepositions	B
—	40. Comprehends simple questions and gives sensible answers	C
NA	56. Can define words	D
NA	57. Uses involved sentences containing: because, but, etc.	D
✓	75. Can execute "triple order," e.g. Put this . . . then . . . and afterwards	E
—	97. Can understand directions: upper left, bottom right, etc.	F
NA	113. Can repeat a story without much difficulty	G

Several items do not apply to the special case of Charles, who is mute. Nevertheless determined teaching and much language support by all staff ought to help in acquiring skills 9 and 97. Considering that he has received a credit on level E (75), it should be fairly easy for him to learn these two skills.

Differences

✓	10. Can tell sex differences (e.g., man, woman, boy, girl)	
✓	27. Can discriminate colours by matching	
NA	41. Differentiates between short, long, big, small, thick, thin	
NA	58. Discriminates and names four or more colours without mistake	
NA	59. Refers correctly to "morning" and "afternoon"	
—	76. Tells "left" and "right" on himself (e.g., left arm, right ear)	
—	77. Names the days of the week and recognises some days	
—	78. Understands difference between: day-week, minute-hour, etc.	
NA	98. Tells the time to a quarter of an hour	
NA	114. Tells the time and associates time on clock with various actions and events	

This child's additional handicap does not permit a straight comparison between his meagre 2 credits and the average attainment of 6 skills. There are, however, 4 skills which are not affected by his muteness and which are probably within his reach - judging by his successes in the following subsections.

Number Work

✓	11. Can differentiate correctly between **one** thing and **many** things	
✓	28. Understands the difference between **two** and **many** things	
NA	42. Can count mechanically ten objects	
✓	43. Can handle "number situations" up to four (including "taking away");	
✓	60. Can arrange objects in order of size from the smallest to the largest	
NA	79. Can count mechanically thirty or more objects	
✓	80. Can handle "number situations" up to 13 or more (including "taking away")	
NA	81. Can recognise coins up to 10p (in the U.S.A. up to a quarter)	
NA	99. Adds coins of various denominations up to 10p (in the U.S.A. up to a quarter)	
✓	115. Can give change out of 10p (in the U.S.A. makes change for a quarter)	

Strict adherence to the Manual criteria penalizes him to some extent and there may well be far more understanding than reflected in the score. A superior performance, despite his handicap, since the 6 credits (when only 4 are expected) are distributed over the whole range A-G.

Paper and Pencil Work

✓	12. Holds pencil and can imitate vertical and circular strokes	
✓	29. Can copy circles	
✓	44. Draws primitive "man" showing head and legs	
✓	61. Draws recognisable "men" and "houses"	
✓	82. Prints his name and recognises it among other printed words and names	
—	83. Can recognise 40 or more words of everyday—or Social Sight Vocabulary (Functional Vocabulary in U.S.A.)	
—	100. "Writes" his name (in script)	
—	101. Reads simple instructions, e.g., on public transport (besides Social Sight Vocabulary)	
✓	102. Addresses envelope in an acceptable manner	
—	116. Reads simple printed matter, e.g., Radio and T.V. Times (Guide)	

Seven credits instead of the expected 4 suggest once again that Charles is probably much brighter than has been assumed. Strenuous efforts should be made to teach him reading since all his deficiencies in this subsection are in this area.

SOCIALISATION

Play Activities

✓ 13.	Plays **in company** with others, but does not yet co-operate with others	A
✓ 30.	Waits "his turn," can "share" at times	B
✓ 45.	Plays co-operatively with others	C
— 46.	Enjoys entertaining others	C
— 62.	Plays competitive games, e.g. hide and seek, tag etc.	D
— 63.	Acts out stories he has heard	D
— 64.	Sings, dances to music, plays records	D
✓ 84.	Plays simple table games, e.g.: tiddly winks, dominoes, snakes and ladders, etc	E
✓ 103.	Plays simple ball games with others, e.g. passing ball	F
✓ 117.	Plays co-operative team games	G

Considering his age, the big gap of missing credits in the middle of this subsection is not very serious. Charles obtains 6 rather than the expected 7 credits, but 3 of them are on a very mature level.

Home Activities

✓ 14.	Fetches and carries on request	A
✓ 31.	Helps in domestic tasks, e.g. clearing table, sweeping, etc.	B
✓ 47.	Goes on simple errands outside the house	C
NO 65.	Is sent into shops or stores, adult waits outside	D
NO 85.	Is trusted with money on errands	E
NO 86.	Goes to one shop or store and purchases specified items	E
✓ 87.	Takes on minor responsibilities	E
NO 104.	Helps at home by going to several shops or stores to fetch specified items	F
✓ 105.	Carries out minor routine tasks without supervision, e.g., emptying waste paper basket, fetching water, milk, newspapers	F
✓ 118.	Does several simple tasks without supervision	G

His performance is better than average. It is disconcerting to see that all 'failures' are due to 'NO'. Charles has been confined to the near home environment (as seen in 94, 11) and this accounts for the 4 'failures'. Further development requires relatively unrestricted access to the immediate neighbourhood.

OCCUPATION

Dexterity (Fine Finger Movements)

✓ 15.	Can string large beads	A
✓ 16.	Can unscrew lids with a twisting movement or turn door knobs	A
— 32.	Can cut paper with scissors	B
✓ 48.	Can make constructive use of plasticine, building blocks, etc.	C
— 49.	Can cut out pictures, though not very accurately	C
✓ 66.	Can wind thread fairly evenly on to a spool	D
✓ 67.	Can build elaborate structures with suitable materials (bricks, construction kits, etc.)	D
— 88.	Can cut cloth with scissors	E
✓ 106.	Can pile papers, playing cards, etc., in a neat way	F
— 119.	Can cut very accurately around outlines	G

Though Charles obtains 7 out of 7 items, analysis of 'failures' indicates quite clearly that he could have obtained a higher score, if he had been taught the use of scissors before reaching school-leaving age.

Agility (Gross Motor Control)

✓ 17.	Can kick ball without falling	A
✓ 33.	Can jump with both feet	B
— 50.	Can stand "tip-toe" for 10 seconds	C
— 68.	Can skip on both feet	D
— 89.	Boys use hammer correctly, girls begin sewing	E
✓ 90.	Can throw ball and hit target (1ft x 1ft), 1½yds away	E
✓ 91.	Uses "playground" apparatus in fairly "safe" and assured manner (swing, see-saw, ropes, etc.)	E
— 107.	Uses tools, kitchen utensils, garden tools	F
— 108.	Can balance on "tip-toe" while bending forward	F
— 120.	Can balance on "tip-toe" in crouched position	G

Again a nearly average performance (5 out of 6). The indications are that Charles could be more competent if he had been encouraged to handly tools of various kinds. He is obviously also rather clumsy and some PE should be useful.

NOTES:

Charles is mute but very responsive. He has lived practically all his life in various institutions. His intellectual abilities gave him IQs between 50 and 60 at different times. His behaviour is quite acceptable at most times. He is being considered for a transfer to a hostel in the open community.

SEE accompanying P-A-C report

> Adhere closely to the criteria
> described in the
> **P-A-C MANUAL**

and written word could be very successful. Making too much
allowance for Charles's muteness will not encourage him suf-
ficiently to tackle new communicative skills. It is regrettable that
Charles's communication skills will have to be tackled in his
adolescence though his competence in numberwork, for example,
should have drawn attention to his relatively high potential whilst
he was still at school.

Charles's home training is very patchy. Despite his willingness to
assist in domestic chores, as evidenced by the good score in 'home
activities', he has not been given sufficient opportunity to assist
indirectly by running errands, etc. (4 NOs). Little emphasis has also
been put on the personal achievements in table habits and washing
skills because the institution has probably neither staff nor time to
insist on the details of domestic living. Too much is done for him
(in order to save time) even though he shows quite some competence in dressing himself adequately.

Altogether 'much room for improvement' as far as the general
teaching approach is concerned. Charles is very likely to benefit
considerably from new opportunities offered in this way.

Note: If this PAC record is the first one of its kind — being
something of a 'school leaver's attainment record', it highlights the
necessity for regular assessments during school time. Such an
assessment would have led to an early intervention to fill in the gaps
in Charles's education. Such a record at the age of sixteen points
also to a general obligation to make up for past omissions by con-
tinuing formal education after the age of 16.

Personal assessment

The diagram of Personal Assessment makes a distinctly lopsided
impression. The very positive valuations of 4 and 5, referring to
various aspects in relationships to other people, represent very
valuable assets to Charles's further career. These attitudes should
help him in 'getting along' and are unlikely to cause friction.

On the other hand the 'dent' in the left top quarter of the
diagram draws attention to some serious shortcomings, the causes
of which have to be investigated. The low rating 2 in 'Independence
in personal care' parallels the poor score in the self-help items of
the social assessment, but is remediable. Some of the unsatisfactory
behaviour shown in the dimensions of 'Adaptation', 'Tempera-
ment', and 'Communicativeness' may derive from feelings of
frustration. The suggested changes in attitude of the staff and the

opening of new vistas to 'outside' may results in more acceptable attitudes in the near future. The poor rating in 'sexual attitude' might reflect the institutional staff's apprehensions regarding interests which are perfectly normal for a sixteen-year-old youth. The criteria for judgment need to be generally formulated, but Charles should be given some help all the same.

THE PRIMARY PROGRESS ASSESSMENT CHART (PPAC)

Case 2

This chart is often used with severely mentally handicapped children. The present case describes an assessment carried out with 'Anne', who was 5 years 3 months old when the assessment was completed.

Compared with other 5-year-old children (mentally handicapped), it appears that generally this child is functioning reasonably well. There is, however, a remarkable superiority in the area of 'communication' and this suggests that other areas, such as 'self-help' and 'occupation' are not only slightly below average, but could perhaps be developed to a much greater degree. The reasons for such disparities need to be investigated in order to establish that low functioning is not due to the absence of opportunities for development, e.g. no stairs. Considering also that the 'dexterity' subsection is so well established, one wonders why associated skills such as 'eating with a spoon' have not been credited. It might be possible that too much help is given unnecessarily. This may be an area which could be tackled first of all in a training programme. There is evidence that much relevant ability is available.

Fig. 3.2.

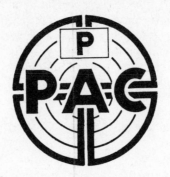

PRIMARY
PROGRESS ASSESSMENT CHART
OF SOCIAL DEVELOPMENT

6th Edition
by
H. C. GÜNZBURG, M.A., Ph.D., F.B.Ps.S.

Acorn Home
(Name of Teaching Centre)

Name: ___ Anne House ___

Address: _____

Date of Birth: 28.2.76   Age 5 y 3m

Date of Assessment: ___ 29.5.81 ___   Signature of Assessor: ___ ⋔ ___

NOTES:

Name: Anne House   Age: 5y 3m

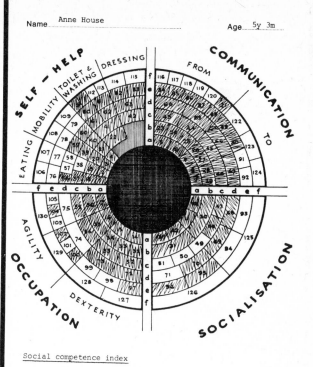

Social competence index

Self help	(26 × 3.45) =	90%
Communication	(28 × 6.25) =	175%
Socialization	(13 × 8.33) =	108%
Occupation	(19 × 4.76) =	90%

Agility (Gross Motor Control)

✓ 16.	Tries to reach objects with hands but overshoots	a
✓ 17.	Manipulates objects	a
✓ 35.	Reaches for objects by leaning forward	b
✓ 36.	Throws objects to floor	b
✓ 54.	Looks for fallen objects by bending over	c
✓ 55.	Aligns two or more cubes or bricks	c
− 74.	Can kick ball without falling	d
− 75.	Throws ball intentionally without falling	d
✓ 100.	Picks up objects without falling	e
− 101.	Can jump with both feet	e
✓ 102.	Opens doors	e
− 103.	Climbs on chair and can stand on it	e
✓ 104.	Seats himself at table	e
− 105.	Takes lid off and puts it back on a box	e
− 129.	Jumps with both feet off bottom step without requiring support	f
− 130.	Stands on one foot for short periods	f

COMMUNICATION—continued

—	117.	Refers to himself as "I"	f
—	118.	Uses question form "Why" . . . .?"	f
—	119.	Expresses feelings, desires, problems verbally	f
—	120.	Able to tell a story, relates experiences in a coherent way	f
✓	121.	Gives full name on request	

To

✓	7.	Listens to music	a
✓	8.	Searches for sound with eyes	a
✓	9.	Turns head to sound	a
✓	26.	Follows moving objects with eyes	b
✓	27.	Looks around him	b
✓	28.	Copies sounds when he hears them	b
✓	29.	Responds to "No"	b
✓	45.	Hands objects on request	c
✓	46.	Responds to questions—e.g. Where is your dress?—if objects are in sight	c
✓	66.	Responds to directions—e.g. Come here	d
✓	67.	Listens to rhythm and is interested in repetition of sounds	d
✓	89.	Obeys simple instructions	e
✓	90.	Listens to simple stories	e
✓	91.	Understands orders containing 'on, in, behind, under, above, in front of, on top of, underneath'	e
—	92.	Can differentiate correctly between **one** thing and **many** things	e
—	122.	Listens to more varied and longer stories	f
—	123.	Listens and can be reasoned with verbally	f
—	124.	Fetches on demand, one or two things. e.g. "give me two books"	f

 SOCIALISATION

✓	10.	Expression shows awareness	a
✓	11.	Reaches, smiles and vocalizes	a
✓	12.	Squirms and responds to people	a
✓	13.	Recognizes familiar people	a
✓	30.	Shows interest in strangers by watching their movements	b
✓	31.	Responds to facial expression, e.g. returns smile	b
✓	47.	Plays 'patacake'	c
✓	48.	Gets attention by making noises	c
—	49.	Wants adult approval for good behaviour	c
	50.	Tries to make others laugh	c
—	51.	Shows affection	d
✓	68.	Looks at mirror image with interest	d
✓	69.	Claims possessions as own	d
✓	70.	Shows objects and offers them	d
—	71.	Waves Bye-Bye	d
—	93.	Plays **in company** with others but does not yet co-operate with others	e
—	94.	Has learnt to respond to other people as they desire	e
—	95.	Fetches and carries on request	e
✓	96.	Is pleased when shown pictures in books	e
—	125.	Waits "his turn", can "share" at times	f
—	126.	Helps in domestic tasks, e.g. clearing table, sweeping, dusting, etc.	f

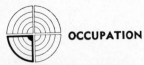 **OCCUPATION**

Dexterity (Fine Finger Movements)

✓	14.	Hands are able to hold objects for short periods	a
✓	15.	Hands are able to grasp objects when offered	a
✓	32.	Transfers things from hand to hand	b
✓	33.	Picks up small objects between finger and thumb	b
✓	34.	Uses index finger to explore	b
✓	52.	Marks with pencil or crayon	c
✓	53.	Puts hand in container, grasps all objects in it	c
✓	72.	Spontaneous scribble with crayon or pencil	d
✓	73.	Puts bricks, boxes, etc., upon another	d
✓	97.	Can string large beads	e
—	98.	Can unscrew lids with a twisting movement, or turn doorknobs	e
—	99.	Pours water from one cup into another	e
—	127.	Can cut paper with scissors	f
—	128.	Handles breakable objects (e.g., crockery) reasonably well	f

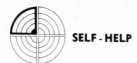

SELF - HELP

Eating

✓	1.	Sucks food well .... a
✓	2.	Shows recognition of food .... a
✓	18.	Puckers his mouth for food .... b
✓	19.	Takes semi-solids from spoon .... b
✓	37.	Uses fingers for eating but does not chew c
✓	38.	Rubs spoon across plate—puts it to mouth for licking c
✓	56.	Chews biscuits, rusks, etc. .... d
—	57.	Prepares edible food by peeling (banana) or unwrapping without reminder being necessary .... d
—	58.	Uses spoon (may spill some food) .... d
—	76.	Drinks from cup unaided without spilling and holds it .... e
—	77.	Eats unaided .... e
—	106.	Uses a fork without difficulty (food can be cut and prepared) .... f
—	107.	Capable of taking a drink by himself without help .... f

Mobility

✓	3.	Balances his head .... a
✓	4.	Sits with slight support .... a
✓	20.	Sits with fairly straight back and without support for short periods .... b
✓	21.	Bounces up and down .... b
✓	39.	Pulls himself upright—stands when holding on c
✓	40.	Gets about by creeping or crawling c
✓	59.	Devises means of getting objects he wants .... d
✓	60.	Walks with aid .... d
NO	78.	Walks upstairs, both feet together on each step .... e
NO	79.	Walks downstairs, both feet together on each step .... e
—	108.	Runs .... f
—	109.	Pushes or pulls large objects .... f

Toilet and Washing

✓	22.	Uses pot (or toilet chair) when placed on it .... b
✓	41.	Bowel movements are generally regular c
✓	61.	Has established some regularity during day time and waits a reasonable time before attended to .... d
✓	62.	Indicates when wet and/or dirty .... d
✓	80.	Bladder control during day, but has to go quite often .... e
✓	81.	"Toilet trained" with infrequent accidents .... e
✓	110.	Asks to go to the toilet or goes by himself .... f
✓	111.	Climbs on lavatory seat .... f
—	112.	Attends to toilet needs without help except for wiping .... f
—	113.	Dries hands adequately without much assistance .... f

Dressing

✓	42.	Co-operates passively when being dressed c
✓	63.	Holds out his arms and feet when being dressed .... d
✓	82.	Assists in getting dressed .... e
✓	83.	Pulls off socks .... e
—	114.	Removes **and** puts on simple articles of clothing .... f
—	115.	Unbuttons accessible buttons .... f

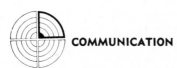

COMMUNICATION

From

✓	5.	Throaty noises, cries .... a
✓	6.	Coos .... a
✓	23.	Mmmm or ssss sounds .... b
✓	24.	Polysyllabic vowels—iii, rrr, etc. .... b
✓	25.	Two syllables—da-da, ba-ba, etc. .... b
✓	43.	One clear word c
✓	44.	Three to four clear words c
✓	64.	Incipient jargon (many intelligible words) .... d
✓	65.	Twenty single words .... d
✓	84.	Two word combinations—daddy go, bye car, etc. .... e
✓	85.	Three word sentences—want a drink, etc. .... e
✓	86.	Pronouns—me, my .... e
✓	87.	Refers to himself by his own name .... e
✓	88.	Uses names of familiar objects .... e
—	116.	Constantly asks questions—What's that? What's this? .... f

THE DEVELOPMENT CHECKLIST

Although the developmental checklist can be used for assessment, its main attraction lies in identifying what therapy targets should be taught *next* in the child's personal development. This checklist is arranged assuming the order in which normal children usually learn things. The checklist is divided into five main sections with different developmental steps for each section. It covers what normal children can do up to approximately five years of age. The authors of this checklist suggest it may be used with mentally handicapped adults. It has also been used effectively with mentally handicapped children. The five sections of the Developmental Checklist are outlined below.

THE DEVELOPMENTAL CHECKLIST

SECTION 1: MOVEMENT

1. Makes crawling movements when lying on stomach.
2. Kicks forcefully.
3. Can bear some weight on legs when held — and lifts foot.
4. Can move head from side to side.
5. Can sit with support — head steady.
6. Can sit in chair briefly.
7. Can bear most weight on legs — when held.
8. Stands with help.
   Sits for one minute or more.
9. Stands holding furniture — cannot lower himself.
   Moves by rolling and squirming on floor.
   Can pull self to sit for 10 minutes.
   Sitting — can lean forward to reach, but not sideways.
10. Pulls and lowers to stand with furniture.
    Sits indefinitely.
11. Walks when led with two hands.
    Walks on hands and feet like a bear.
    Sitting — can twist round to pick up things.
12. Stands alone for a few seconds.
    Walks round furniture and walks when led with one hand.
    Crawls rapidly.
    Can rise to sitting from lying.

13. Walks unsteadily and gets to feet alone.
    Can rise from sitting to standing without support.
    Climbs stairs on hands and knees.
    Kneels without support.
14. Walks well.
    Walks up and down stairs with help.
    Stoops and picks up things from floor without falling.
    Can seat self on chair.
    Can make a few steps sideways and backwards.
15. Runs on whole foot.
    Jumps with both feet.
    Walks up and down stairs — two feet on each step.
    Squats when playing — stands without using hands.
    Pulls chair up to table.
16. Can walk on tiptoe.
    Can cross feet or knees when sitting.
17. Goes upstairs, one foot on each step.
18. Goes downstairs, one foot on each step.
    Hops.
    Picks up objects from floor — bends at waist.
    Marches in time to music.
19. Can walk along a straight line.
    Skips.
    Runs well.

SECTION 2: SOCIAL SKILLS (GETTING ON WITH OTHERS)

NOTE: *You may not want to teach the items in brackets in the following lists, but they are included because they occur during normal development.*

1. Smiles at others when they approach him.
   Quietens when picked up.
   Watches mother when feeding.
2. Smiles and makes noises when talked to.
3. Smiles back at smiling face.
   Shows interest in surroundings — looks around and makes noises.
   Recognizes mother — smiles, makes noises, etc. when he sees her.
4. Smiles at people before they approach him.
   Friendly to strangers.
5. Stops crying when talked to.

   6. Holds out arms to be picked up.
      Responds to emotional tone of mother's voice.
      Knows who are strangers (e.g. frowns and stares at them).
   9. (Needs reassurance before accepting advances of strangers.)
  10. (Pulls mother's clothes for attention.)
  12. (Demonstrates affection for familiar people.)
      May kiss when asked to.
  13. (Moods change quickly.)
  14. (Dislikes being left.)
      (Demands a lot of attention.)
  15. Plays near but not with other children.
      Plays happily alone, but likes to be with adult.
      Follows adult around.
      (Tantrums when he doesn't get his own way — easily stopped.)
  16. Watches other children playing — occasionally joins in for a time.
      (Violent tantrums when he doesn't get his own way.)
  17. Joins in play with other children.
      Creates own play — plays on his own happily for some time.
      Recognizes sex differences: tells you who is a boy, who is a girl.
      Separates from mother easily.
      (Affectionate and confiding.)
      Able to tidy up toys if encouraged.
      Shares toys, sweets, etc.
  18. Takes turns.
      Plays in small group of children.
      Performs for others, e.g. recites, dances, etc.
      Goes on short distance errands, e.g. to neighbours.
      (General behaviour self-willed.)
      (Needs friends of his own age.)
  19. Follows group rules.
      Plays competitive exercise games.
      (Tantrums much less frequent.)
      (Chooses own friends.)

SECTION 3: SELF HELP

Eating and drinking

   1. Sucks well.
   2. Shows anticipation when about to be fed.
   5. Pats bottle.
      Holds bottle.
   6. Drinks from cup when held to lips.
      Holds spoon with help.
      Sucks soft food off spoon.
      Chews and eats biscuit when fed with it.

7. Keeps lips closed when offered more food than he wants.
9. Helps to hold cup for drinking.
   Feeds self with biscuit.
   Rubs spoon across plate.
10. (Finger feeds.)
12. Drinks from cup with a little help.
    Holds spoon — cannot use it alone.
13. Manages cup up and down without much spilling.
    Holds spoon, brings to mouth and licks, but spoon tends to rotate.
    Chews well — some mess.
    Can manage to eat food on his own, but messily.
14. Uses cup with both hands.
    Spoon no longer rotates.
    Hands empty dish to mother.
    Discriminates edible substances (doesn't eat rubbish, may bite objects, but no need to watch him).
15. Uses cup with one hand — no spilling.
    Pours from one cup to another.
    Uses spoon competently.
    Chews competently.
    Removes wrapper from sweet before eating.
16. Sucks through straw.
    Gets drink unassisted, e.g. water, milk.
    Uses fork — not very well.
17. Pours from jug.
    Eats with spoon and fork — messy.
    Handles breakable objects.
18. Eats skilfully with spoon and fork.
    Beginning to use knife and fork.
19. Uses knife and fork.
    Spreads with knife.
    Prepares simple foods, e.g. jelly.

Toiletting and washing

3. Enjoys bath.
10. Shows discomfort when wet or soiled.
12. Gives some indication of need for toilet.
    Plays with flannel and toys in the bath.
13. Regularity — usually urinates when sat on pot or toilet at a regular time.
    Sometimes asks for pot or toilet.
14. Dry by day, occasional accidents.
    (Urgency over urine passing.)
15. Tells you his toilet needs in reasonable time.
    Goes to toilet by self for bowels.
    Dry at night if lifted in the evening.
    Attempts to soap and wash self in the bath.

16. Goes to toilet by self for urine.
    Pulls off pants at toilet — seldom replaces.
    Climbs on to toilet seat.
    Inadequate attempt to wash hands.
    Dries hands acceptably if reminded.
17. Attends to toilet needs without help except for wiping.
    Dry by night.
    Dries hands well.
18. Attends to toilet needs fully — wipes, washes and dries hands well.
    Brushes teeth.
19. Washes face well.
    Washing, apart from face and hands, requires help.
    Tidies hair occasionally.

Dressing
11. Holds out arm for sleeve, or foot for shoe.
12. Takes off socks.
    Helps with dressing — holding out limbs.
13. Takes off shoes.
14. Unzips.
15. Takes off pants, coat and dress. (May be unfastened for him.)
    Puts on shoes, socks, and pants.
16. Unbuttons front buttons.
17. Undresses fully except back fastenings.
    Puts on coat.
    Attempts to fasten button.
    Partially dresses self if reminded.
18. Dresses and undresses except for back fastenings.
    Can fasten buttons.
    Puts on vest and tight T-shirt.
19. Laces shoes and ties laces.
    Dresses and undresses without help.

SECTION 4: PLAY

Looking at things and colours
(The four primary colours are red, blue, green, and yellow. Matching a colour means putting something of one colour with something of the same colour — nothing need be said.)

1. Eyes follow object dangling in front of face. Looks at face briefly.
2. Eyes follow a moving person.
3. Eyes follow object moving from side to side. Looks at own hands intently.
   Eyes focus on near object.
   Looks steadily at faces.
4. Looks at dropped object.
5. Looks at object on table.
   Smiles at himself in mirror.
6. Eyes move in unison (no longer stares at hands).

7. Pats image of himself in mirror.
   Will change his position to see an object not in front of him.
9. Looks for an object hidden while watching.
10. Looks round a corner for object.
11. Points at objects through glass.
12. Looks for and finds an object hidden before his eyes.
14. Points at distant objects out of doors.
16. Matches one primary colour.
17. Matches two primary colours.
18. Matches four primary colours.
    Names four primary colours.
19. Names ten colours.
    Names six colours.
    Matches different shapes.

Handling things

2. Holds rattle for a very short time.
3. Grasps hold of an object when it is placed in his hand.
   Shakes rattle for a very short time.
   Plays with own hands.
4. Shakes rattle for long periods of time.
5. Will grasp objects on his own.
   Pats objects.
   Uses either hand to reach for objects.
6. Reaches for objects.
   Can transfer objects from one hand to the other.
   When drops objects, forgets them.
7. Shakes rattle hard.
   Bangs objects on table.
   Usually uses preferred hand to reach for objects (i.e. he is right-handed or left-handed).
8. Strikes objects with other objects.
   Pulls string to get an object.
9. Pokes objects with index finger (first finger).
   Picks objects up with index finger and thumb instead of whole hand.
   Throws objects on floor on purpose.
   Offers object to you, but will not let it go.
10. Reaches for toys and explores them with his hands.
12. Throws objects on floor again and again.
    Gives objects to you when you ask — sometimes gives them without you asking.
13. Picks up small objects neatly.
14. Uses a stick to get an object that is out of his reach.
15. Is definitely right-handed or left-handed.
16. Folds a piece of paper in half. Can move fingers separately.
18. Cuts paper into 3 equal squares.
19. Can sew roughly.
    Can tie a knot at the end of thread.
    Makes models with playdough or plasticene.

Cubes, bricks, formboards, and puzzles

(A formboard is a tray with pieces you can take out. A puzzle is cut-up pieces that you can put together.)

6. If he is holding one cube, will drop it when you offer him another.
7. If he is holding one cube will hold on to it when you offer him another.
9. Holds 2 cubes with both hands.
12. Puts cubes in a box.
13. Holds 2 cubes in one hand.
    Builds a 2-cube tower.
    Puts round block in round hole in formboard.
14. Builds a 4-cube tower.
    Puts round and square blocks in round and square holes in formboard.
15. Does simple 3-piece formboard.
    Puts large pegs in peg-board.
16. Builds an 8-cube tower.
    Does 2-piece jigsaw puzzle.
17. Builds a 10-cube tower.
    Does 3-4-piece jigsaw puzzle.
18. Copies a 3-cube pyramid. (That is, if you build one first, he will copy yours.)
    Builds simple things with *Lego*.
    Does 4-8-piece jigsaw puzzle.
19. Plans and builds constructively (builds house with *Lego*).
    Does 12-piece jigsaw puzzle.

Books, paper, crayons, and scissors

5. Crumples paper in hands.
12. Looks at pictures in book.
    Holds crayon or pencil in fist.
13. Pats picture in book.
    Helps turn pages.
    Copies straight scribble.
14. Enjoys simple picture book.
    Will point to coloured parts of picture when you ask (for example, 'Show me the ball').
    Turns several pages together.
    Scribbles using preferred hand (he is right-handed, or left-handed).
15. Turns pages one by one.
    Will point to detailed items when you ask (e.g., 'Show me the girl's hair'.)
    Copies vertical and circular scribble.
16. Copies horizontal scribble.
    Beginning to draw on his own.
    Folds paper.
    Holds scissors clumsily — beginning to cut.

17. Draws a man with head and one other part.
    Paints with large brush and easel.
    Cuts out pictures — not very accurately.
18. Matches pictures.
    Copies a cross.
    Uses scissors with ease.
    Draws a simple house.
19. Copies a triangle and letters.
    Draws a recognizable man.
    Using scissors — can cut along a line.
    Can cut cloth.

Action toys, screwing and threading toys

12. Pushes little cars.
    Rolls ball to adult.
13. Pushes large wheeled toys.
    Rolls ball on his own.
14. Strings cotton reels.
15. Throws and kicks ball.
    Strings large beads (one inch).
    Throws ball into basket.
16. Turns door-knobs and screws lids.
17. Plays on the floor with cars, bricks, etc.
    Climbs nursery apparatus well.
    Uses pedal on tricycle.
    Strings small beads (half an inch).
18. Climbs ladders and trees.
    Catches large ball.
19. Uses slides and swings.
    Can use hammer.
    Can wind fairly evenly on to a spool.
    Uses screwdriver.
    Can use saw.

Copying and pretending

1. Looks at faces for a short while.
   Stares at mother's face when she is talking to or feeding him.
2. Smiles and makes noises when talked to.
3. Looks at surroundings with interest.
   Focuses eyes on a near object.
   Looks at object in front of him straight away.
   Shows anticipation when about to be fed or lifted (for example, opens
   his mouth when he sees food, holds out his arms when mother holds
   out hers).
4. Pulls dress over face.
5. Smiles at himself in mirror.
6. Laughs when his head is hidden (for example, under a towel).
   Copies you if you cough or stick your tongue out at him.

7. Copes very simple acts and noises (for example, arm waving, 'goo-gooing').
   Enjoys 'peepbo', but does not yet play himself.
   Pats image of himself in mirror.
8. Copies you shaking a rattle, ringing a bell, etc.
9. Copies hand-clapping.
10. Plays 'pat-a-cake'.
    Waves 'bye-bye' when shown.
12. Plays 'peepbo' covering his face.
    Knows what body movement is coming next when nursery rhymes are said.
    Plays up and down games.
13. Begins to copy mother doing housework.
14. Briefly copies simple action (for example, kissing a doll, reading a book).
    Copies mother washing, dusting, and cleaning.
15. Pretending play begins (for example, making a toy animal walk).
    Plays copying mother's domestic tasks (for example, putting a doll to bed).
17. Can copy closing first and wiggling thumb.
18. Strong dramatic play and dressing-up (for example, being a nurse).
    Sometimes has a pretend friend.
19. Acts stories out in detail.

SECTION 5: LANGUAGE

Understanding

1. Watches mother closely when she speaks.
3. Turns towards a nearby voice or meaningful sound.
   Shows distress through a loud sound.
4. Excites on hearing steps; that is, he makes noises and movements.
   Looks straight at bell, rattle, etc., when he hears it.
   Responds to emotional tone of mother's voice (for example, cries when she sounds cross, laughs when she sounds happy).
8. Stops what he is doing for a short while when you say 'No'.
9. Listens to wristwatch or clock.
10. Responds to some words (for example, looks or points when you say 'Where's Daddy?').
12. Immediately turns to his own name.
    Understands and obeys simple commands with gesture (for example, 'Give me . . .', 'Wave bye-bye').
    Comes when called.
    Goes to points directed.
13. Understands and obeys simple commands without gesture (for example, 'Shut the door'; 'Give me the ball'; 'Get your shoes').
    Points to familiar persons, toys, etc. when asked.
14. Follows directions (for example, 'Put the doll on the chair').
    Shows own or doll's hair, shoes, etc. when asked.
    Pictures — points to one named thing.

15. Points to five parts of doll or self.
    Shows 3 objects or pictures when asked.
    (Prepositions are words like *in, on, under, behind, beside,* etc.)
    Can carry out two different prepositions when you ask him (for example, 'Put the cup *under* the table', 'Put the car *in* the box').
16. Shows you objects when you describe them by their use (for example, 'What do we cut with?').
    If asked to pass *one,* does not pass more.
17. Listens to short story.
    Gives two out of many.
18. Can carry out for different prepositions when asked.
    Can show you which is the longer of two lines.
    Can show you which is the big one and the small one of two objects (for example, two cups).
19. Can carry out a triple order preposition (for example, 'Put the spoon *in* the cup, put the cup *under* the table and then sit *on* the chair').

Speech — general conversation

1. Makes throaty noises.
   'Coos' when happy.
2. Says 'Ah, eh, oh'.
3. Says most vowel sounds, 'Ah, eh, oh, uh, ih'.
4. Laughs aloud.
5. Says 'Ahgoo'.
6. Grunts and growls.
   Says single and double syllables.
   Screams when annoyed.
7. Says 'da, ka, ba, ga'.
8. Says 'dada, baba'.
9. Babbles (syllables, not words).
   Shouts to attract attention.
10. Shakes head for 'No'.
12. Asks for objects by pointing.
    Tries to sing.
13. Speaks 2-6 words.
    Uses gesture to make his wants known.
    Uses one word to cover several words (e.g. 'dada' is all men).
14. Speaks 6-20 words.
    Echoes prominent or last word said to him.
15. Speaks 50+ words.
    Echoes many words.
    Talks continuously to himself when playing.
    Speaks his food and toilet needs.
    Speaks 2-word sentences.
16. Speaks 200+ words.
    Uses pronouns: I, me, you.
    Combines two ideas (for example, 'Daddy gone', 'More chocolate').
    Uses plurals.
    Says 3-word sentences.

17. Carries on simple conversation.
    Asks what, where, who.
    Says 4-word sentences.
18. Uses conjunctions like: and, but, so, etc.
19. Can tell you a connected account of recent things that have happened to him.

Speech — answers to questions

 8. Copies sounds (for example, 'ooh, uuh').
12. Copies animal noises that you make (for example, 'meow, woof').
    Tries to copy words.
15. Gives first name.
    Shows and repeats hair, eyes, shoes, etc.
    Names 2-3 objects in picture book.
    Names 3-5 objects.
17. Gives full name and sex.
    May count up to 10 (without objects to count).
    Answers simple questions (for example, 'What did you have for breakfast?').
    Repeats two numbers you say to him (for example '6, 8').
18. Gives address and age.
    Counts three objects placed in front of him.
    Listens to and tells simple stories.
    Can repeat three numbers you say to him (for example, 3, 9, 2').
    Can explain simple concepts, like toys, animals, food, etc. (for example, 'You can eat food', 'Toys are things you play with').
    Can tell you what to do when hungry, cold, etc. (for example, 'When you are cold, you put on your coat').
    Can tell you what day of the week it is.
    Enjoys jokes.
    Can tell you what simple things are made of (for example, table of wood).
19. Gives birthday.
    Counts five fingers on one hand.
    Can tell you whether it is morning or afternoon.
    Repeats four numbers you say to him.
    Defines some simple words (for example, 'A ball is round, it bounces, and you play with it'; 'A dog is an animal with four legs which barks').
    Can name days of the week in order.
    Can tell you which is longer of day/week, hour/minute, etc.
    Can tell you the month and the year.
    Tells left and right on himself.

The authors of the Developmental Checklist give some helpful advice on scoring the list. This should be studied in detail by each nurse and adhered to when practising assessment and therapy.

However, a number of practical points are summarized here to give the nurse an idea of how the checklist might be used.

Guidelines for using the Developmental Checklist

1. Tick or make a clear mark such as a plus sign next to the behaviours the child can carry out.
2. Observe the child closely when completing the checklist.
3. Where the child does not show the behaviour under assessment do *not* give a 'pass' for that area of development.
4. Where the child fails to perform a checklist behaviour because of a physical handicap 'H' should be marked next to that item.
5. Where the child is credited with behaviours advanced on the checklist, in many cases it suggests previous steps have been mastered. Walking is an example. Where children can walk it can be assumed that they have passed the previous items on the movement scale.
6. A cautious and critical attitude should however be maintained by any nurse using this checklist. For there may be occasions when the passes advanced on the checklist do not imply attainment of behaviour earlier on in the section of the checklist. For instance in handling things during play, the child may shake a rattle vigorously but not yet transfer an object from one hand to the other.
7. When all of the sections of the checklist have been completed, transfer the results of the assessment to the teaching chart (see Fig. 3.3). Doing this helps to show clearly and graphically the overall and detailed developmental profile of the child under assessment.
8. It is a useful practice to colour in or number the assessment which has just been completed. This serves to show the areas of development achieved by the child and those yet to be attained.
9. Leave blank those items the child has not yet performed.
10. Review the assessment with all the relevant people involved with the child (e.g. mother, father, nurse, teacher, social workers, occupational therapist, speech therapist, psychologist) and identify the things in his development he would benefit from learning next.

11.　Where possible, select behaviour which each mentally handi-
　　capped child or adolescent is likely to be able to learn, and
　　which will contribute to their balanced development.

TEACHING CHART

Colour in each step the child can do. Do not colour it in if the child cannot
do all the items in that step.

If the child cannot do a step because of physical handicap, write H.

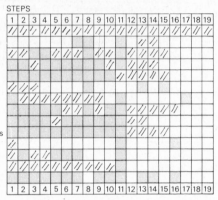

STEPS

	1	2	3	4	5	6	7	8	9	10	11	12	13	14	15	16	17	18	19
MOVEMENT																			
SOCIAL SKILLS (Getting on with others)																			
SELF HELP: Drinking and eating																			
Toiletting and washing																			
Dressing																			
PLAY: Looking at things and colours																			
Handling things																			
Cubes, bricks, formboards, and puzzles																			
Books, paper, crayons, and scissors																			
Action toys, screwing and threading toys																			
Copying and pretending																			
LANGUAGE: Understanding																			
Speech – general conversation																			
Speech – answers to questions	1	2	3	4	5	6	7	8	9	10	11	12	13	14	15	16	17	18	19

NAME: John C.　AGE: 9 y 4 m

Fig. 3.3.

Case 3

Figure 3.3 shows how the Developmental Checklist can be used with
a mentally handicapped child. 'John' was aged 9 years 4 months at
the time of his assessment. The checklist was completed during his
school hours. The checklist chart reveals the overall profile of
John's current level of development. It is patchy and indicates
areas where therapy targets might be selected to promote further
development. The 'hatched' lines across each developmental
section highlight this quite clearly. Each of the areas of
development shown in Fig, 3.3 are transferred from an assessment
of different behaviours in the developmental checklist. The checklist is also used to identify therapy targets which are drawn from the
overall assessment. 'John's' report was compiled in the following
way:

Report

John suffered meningitis when he was one year old and his mother
says his problems started then. He has been labelled 'autistic' and is
now in a school for autistic children. He spends most of his time

rushing about, does not play constructively, has little eye-contact and very little language, either receptive or spoken. Assessment took place over a two-week period when John was observed daily. Assessment involved not only observation, but physically assisting John to sit in order to carry out some of the tasks.

Targets drawn from assessment

Sitting at table for 2 minutes.
Requirements for therapy: (1) looking at therapist when name is called; (2) looking at objects on 'task' table.

Checklist targets for therapy

   (1)   Smiling at others;
   (2)   imitating simple actions; and
   (3)   turning to direction of noises.

Note in this case, in addition to an assessment, therapy targets are drawn from the checklist. It will be shown later how the nurse can proceed with assessment and the identification of therapy targets to be learnt. The case example from the Developmental Checklist also illustrates neatly how *clear* behavioural targets can be selected for incorporating into any therapy plan. The clearer the therapy targets, the less ambitious the task will be for nurses to put the therapy plans into practice. Clear and consistent assessment is essential for behaviour therapy to take place. When more than one therapist is employing therapy with a mentally handicapped child, it is of primary importance to check that they do *not* differ in their assessment of that child. One way of avoiding this difficulty is to become familiar with each developmental scale (reading the scale manuals were appropriate), and using them in practice.

Using developmental scales and checklists

Broadly speaking, the developmental scales and checklists have been constructed from knowledge of the psychology of normal child development. They also include work which has been done on the development of mentally handicapped people. Although these scales are not ideal for all assessments, they provide a valuable starting-point in the approach to therapeutic nursing. Their strengths and weaknesses will become apparent when it comes to drawing up a plan of therapy. Where this happens it should be looked upon as an opportunity to evaluate, and if necessary, alter the therapist's approach to assessment. These occasions should also be seen as useful opportunities for asking a clinical psychologist to share in the discussion and the solving of problems. However, the main areas of assessment where the nurse should work most closely with the psychologist are the skills and behaviours the developmental charts set out to measure. There are six categories of development common to most of the charts listed.

Main categories of development measured on developmental charts

1. *Motor development — movement*. Assessing whether or not the child can use his own body, e.g. walking, climbing. Also, what he knows about it, e.g. where his nose, mouth, eyes, etc. are.
2. *Self-help skills*. Also known as self-care skills. Finding out if the child can do things for himself, e.g. feeding, dressing, toiletting, etc.
3. *Social skills*. Assessing the state of personal relationships between the child and other people, e.g. sharing behaviour, holding a short conversations, etc.
4. *Play*. Assesses at what level of play the child is functioning, e.g. imitating, copy-play, make-believe, inventing own games, etc. Also provides some idea of how the child learns.
5. *Language*. Assesses current language skills, e.g. number of words/sounds babble; one-word, two-word sentences; imitation, word play.
6. *Communication*. Assesses whether communication is mainly by language or gestures, or both. Also whether language precedes action, or action precedes language.

There is one other category which should be added to this list. It is not included in some charts, but deserves mention because of the prevalence of so-called problem behaviour in mentally handicapped children.

7. *Socially desirable behaviour*. Which behaviours are desirable as determined by society, e.g. behaviour which is harmful to themselves or others — biting, scratching, gouging, etc.

Where it is not appropriate to use developmental charts, it will be important for nurses to construct forms which permit accurate recording of behaviours which are not socially desirable. These should also be used for observation and assessment of *desirable* behaviour. We often overlook the degree of desirable social behaviour expressed by the mentally handicapped and instead tend to emphasize undesirable aspects of their behaviour.

When the assessment phase has taken place a Personal Assessment Profile (PAP) should be drawn up for each child. Collaboration with a clinical psychologist specializing in mental handicap should prove helpful in identifying therapy targets. Therapy targets are identified by employing the tools of assessment in a consistent and methodical way. The nurse must, therefore, practise a disciplined approach to assessment. Each chart has its own guide or manual of the assessment method and techniques to be used. For any assessment to be valid and have therapeutic value, the guides and manuals must be read, understood, and used in practice. There are however, a number of assessment rules to observe which are common to many developmental charts.

General rules of assessment

Each scale has its own items of behaviour to be assessed. If the child being assessed does perform the behaviour the nurse is looking for (e.g. brushes own teeth, washes own hands, looks at own face in mirror), then a tick or check mark should be entered on the chart next to that item. If the child does not perform the behaviour under assessment, leave the chart blank. Where the child has had no opportunity to demonstrate the behaviour under assessment, either leave the chart blank or give some indication of the opportunity restrictions imposed by the assessment circumstances (e.g. indicating this by 'NO'). A similar approach should be adopted for items that are not applicable (e.g. marking these items 'NA').

In practice, it is not always easy to be consistent. Nurses may find themselves saying, 'He can do it when he wants to', 'He can do it sometimes', or 'She can't quite do it yet, but . . .'. Whenever this happens and it is not clear if the person being assessed has learnt a specific behaviour, there is an assessment rule to apply. There are many rules of assessment, but there are three main ones which the nurse-therapist should observe:

1. *Do not credit a mentally handicapped child with something they cannot do.*
2. *Do not credit a mentally handicapped child with something they may be able to do, but have not had the opportunity of doing.*

3. *Do credit a mentally handicapped child for the things you see them doing most of the time.*

The reason for adopting this disciplined approach to assessment is in the interests of the mentally handicapped child and the assessor. Crediting a mentally handicapped child with something they do not regularly do, gives a false impression of their level of learning. In turn, this error leads to wrong and often overoptimistic choices of what to teach the child, and what therapy to plan. If we look at therapy as teaching the mentally handicapped to learn more complex behaviour, the difficulties we can create for them will become apparent. For, in many ways, the mentally handicapped child is a child who is slow to learn complex behaviours. If we choose behaviours for therapy which are too complex, we are making it doubly difficult for them to learn. It is also probable that learning new and excessively complex behaviours in therapy will not be enjoyable for them. This principle applies to all kinds of behaviour. Creating learning tasks outside the learning ability of the child may also lead to frustration for them. Learning behaviours in this way may well become a punishing experience. Assessment must therefore be realistic and governed by the rules of assessment for therapy planning and effective therapeutic practice. Another trap to avoid is eagerly moving on to teaching another behaviour in therapy, when the first target behaviour has not been established. The mentally handicapped child needs to establish learning in self-help skills, play, communication, and social behaviour before embarking on more ambitious projects. There are two further practical guidelines to adopt which help to avoid difficulties later in therapy.

1. *Repeat skills which are known to the mentally handicapped child many times.*
2. *Build up the child's confidence before moving on to teach more difficult behaviour.*

It is just as important not to assume that, because a mentally handicapped child can do some of the tasks on a developmental scale, he must be able to do other things on that scale, e.g. because he can wash his hands he should be able to wash his cup. Similarly, because a mentally handicapped child can attend to his personal hygiene in hospital, it does not necessarily mean he can do it in his own parents' home. Assessment should always examine the assumption that a mentally handicapped child is *able* to produce the *same behaviour* in *different situations*. Because of the wide range of handicapping conditions and, more so, the individual learning rate and learning style of the mentally handicapped, the assessment of abilities, learning, and behaviour, should be personalized and individual. The developmental scales are only guides to assessment. However, they are useful practical guides when used consistently. They provide clear behaviours that might be learnt by the mentally handicapped child. They do not however show us the way in which therapy might proceed. This topic is taken up in Chapter 8 where therapy techniques are discussed.

ASSIGNMENT 1

Assessment

1. Select a child or adolescent who has not had a previous assessment.

2. Using an appropriate developmental scale or checklist carry out a developmental assessment as a team.

3. Each person in the team should carry out a complete assessment (for instance if there are three members in a team, three assessments of the same child or adolescent should be carried out). Therapy targets should *not* be identified at this stage.

4. When the assessments have been completed, come together as a team and discuss, under supervision, areas of agreement and disagreement about the assessments you have completed.

5. As a team now identify therapy targets to be incorporated in a therapy plan. The targets should specify clearly the behaviours you agree the child or adolescent should learn in order to promote fulfilment of his psychological needs.

6. Draw up and define the actions you have taken as a team. Outline the use of the developmental scale or checklist and the reasons why it was adopted. State clearly why your team selected their particular behaviours that they wanted the child to learn.

7. Compile a report of the assessment assignment and present it to your supervisor for discussion with your team.

ASSIGNMENT 2

Assessment

1. Carry out an assignment as above but as an individual.
2. Compile a report of the assessment assignment and present it to your supervisor for discussion.

4

Observation

THE IMPORTANCE OF OBSERVATION

One of the greatest difficulties which can crop up in assessing mentally handicapped children is deciding whether or not they have learned a particular skill or new behaviour. One helpful way of increasing confidence in any assessment is to confirm it by adequate observation. Observation provides the evidence on which solid assessments of a child's behaviour and development can be made. The mentally handicapped, like their normal contemporaries, do not always do what we want them to do when we think they should do it. For the purposes of assessment it is important to help the mentally handicapped child to like learning. To achieve this we must first find out what they already enjoy doing and what they do not enjoy doing. Another less subjective way of looking at observation is to establish those behaviours which the child engages in a great deal and those which are infrequent or absent. This means observing the child in a number of different settings and at different times in those settings. It also involves using the observations made by parents, nurses, social workers, psychologists, speech therapists, occupational therapists, physiotherapists and so on. Using valid observational information for each child is essential to assessment and the planning of nursing therapy. For instance, if we assess a child to find out at what times in the day he learns new behaviour quickest, we may find he learns best immediately after breakfast. Another child may be sleepy and distractible immediately after breakfast, and at his best for learning new behaviours in the afternoon. Important facts like these can only be assessed by close systematic observation and consultation with a wide range of personnel involved with any particular child. The basis for therapy planning springs from the *evidence* of assessment and observation.

LOOKING AND SEEING

Observing and looking at people is something we do every day of our lives. When we look we usually use our eyes and when we observe we use our eyes and some of the other senses — hearing, smell, touch, etc. In observing mentally handicapped children however, we should employ a systematic set of procedures for observation. All such observational approaches should specify in advance what it is that is to be observed and how it is to take place, e.g. picking up a spoon: how many times a spoon is lifted; or in problem behaviour (biting, scratching, punching): how often it occurs in different situations. By employing this systematic approach, it become possible to derive a detailed profile of the behaviour under assessment and observation. Nurses should also increase their awareness of what *they* are *doing* during observation periods, and how they go about observing mentally handicapped children. This also means sharing with their colleagues what they are doing when they are observing and how they are carrying out their observations.

In all the observational efforts employed by nurses, they should be actively looking out for the behaviours they want to increase, and those behaviours they want to decrease. Broadly speaking, this means trying to find out at least five things during observation.

1. *Where* the behaviour is shown, e.g. cloakroom, playground, television room, school classroom, lavatory, home-kitchen, own room, etc.
2. *When* the child shows specific behaviour under assessment, e.g. Monday 10 a.m.-10.10 a.m.
3. *Who* and *what* is present when the behaviour is shown, e.g. parents, psychologist, nurse, food, toys, etc.
4. *How often* the behaviour occurs, e.g. 1, 7, 15 times per day, less than 5 times every 10 minutes, more than 10 times every 10 minutes.
5. *What happens before* and *immediately after* the behaviour occurs, e.g. toy taken away and given back again, breakfast arrived, breakfast given to child.

Disciplined recording of these kinds of observations should provide the nurse with a basis for analysing the behaviour they are observing. This means that in, say, observing self-care skills or problem behaviours, we should derive a picture of what maintains such behaviour. Included in the same analysis of these observations are often clues as to how behaviour might be changed. In other words we should also get a clear idea of *why* mentally handicapped children behave the way they do.

SOME METHODS OF OBSERVING

There are many methods used by psychologists to observe behaviour under assessment. However, there are two which are most likely to be used by nurses. These are:

1. *Time sampling.* The simplest example of time sampling is recording exactly how often a specified behaviour is occurring in a given period of time, e.g. every five minutes. Using observation periods to record painting boxes, folding clothes, head-banging, etc.
2. *Episode observation.* Typical episode observations involve recording (whenever possible) every instance of a particular behaviour's taking place, e.g. biting, head-banging, soiling, temper tantrums, washing hands, and so on. These observations may also record when the child expresses the behaviour, and where and who is present when it occurs.

The type of observation method used should be determined by the behaviour the nurse wishes to assess. It should also be determined by the therapy goals the nurse has worked out with colleagues and the clinical psychologist for a particular child or group. The main point the nurse should keep in mind is to find out as much as possible *first* about the child *before* proceeding with therapy. This is one of the cardinal principles of observation and assessment. It is usually called the baseline measurement or more generally, the baseline period.

BASELINE PERIOD

During the baseline period, baseline recordings are made of a wide range of behaviours on the lines of those shown on the developmental checklists. These are then used to assess and analyse what behaviours to reduce, promote, expand, and what priorities should be given to therapy targets. Highly specific behaviours may also be recorded during the baseline period. These can often involve baseline recording of the so-called problem behaviours — kicking, biting, scratching, hair-pulling, and self-mutilation.

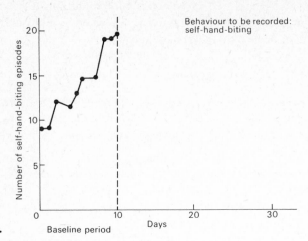

Fig. 4.1.   Baseline period

Recording baselines (see Fig. 4.1) before therapy allows the nurse to compare the person's behaviour after therapy has begun with their original behaviour. In this way, the nurse is able to answer questions like (a) have the targets behaviours selected for therapy been relevant for this particular handicapped person?; (b) was the therapy employed in the way it was planned?; and (c) did the therapy employed achieve the targets set? The answers to these questions will show whether or not the nurse has designed, carried out, and achieved 'good' therapy.

In order to discover what makes a mentally handicapped child learn and how to help him succeed in learning new behaviour, it is essential to *carry out systematic assessment and observations.* This must be done accurately for assessment and observation to have any therapeutic value. In the home, mental handicap hospital, and special school, there is an overdue need to make *all* personnel aware of the crucial role assessment and observation play in therapy.

The three main reasons for keeping baseline records of observations can be summarized:

1. They help all personnel involved with a mentally handicapped child to get a clear and concise set of systematic assessment details about him. A practical example of this use is in the changeover from day to night-shift of nursing staff. By using baseline records each shift will have the same information and avoid confusion over their 'assessment' of any particular child.

The same applies when a mentally handicapped child moves from one location to another, for example, moves from his own home to a foster home, or changes schools.

2. They help to provide assessment evidence on which therapy plans are formulated.

3. They also help nurses and other appointed therapists to evaluate the success of therapy plans when they are put into practice.

RECORDING OBSERVATIONS

Practical pointers

1. Remember to complete any important factual information and personal history such as names, date of birth, date assessment commenced and finished, relevant diagnosis, etc. A great deal of relevant information can be obtained from existing records and working with other sources, e.g. psychologist, speech therapist, parents.

2. The observations which have to be recorded in any assessment should be kept in mind during the day. This should help nurses to 'look' for the selected behaviour under assessment. In this way, a few assessment observations can be completed each day. Employing this kind of approach permits assessment to progress in 'natural' way, e.g. toiletting behaviour can be assessed at the time the child usually goes to the lavatory. The same applies to recording observations of feeding behaviour and other self-catering skills. The exception to this method is those behaviours which do not occur at predictable times, e.g. the so-called 'problem' behaviours.

3. Try to choose times which are suitable for both nurse and child. For instance, it is often unwise to start recording observations when the child is unwell, sleepy, or unco-operative (unless behaviours connected with these states are under assessment). Nurses should also plan the amount of time they should allocate to any particular assessment. This can be done in consultation with colleagues such as parents, nurses, teachers, social workers, and the clinical psychologist specializing in the psychology of mental handicap.

4. It is advisable to carry out most observations under or as near 'normal' conditions as possible, e.g. be careful not to give extra attention to the child just because they are being observed. This

is a practical skill which nurses should cultivate with practice. Being an unobtrusive observer reduces the risks of changing the behaviour that is under assessment.

Identifying new and desirable behaviours to promote in the learning of the child is the aim of all assessment and observations. But in the first instance, we should attempt only to complete an accurate baseline assessment by systematically recording the observations made. After this phase of the therapeutic strategy, there should then be sufficient evidence from the assessment to formulate a therapy plan.

ASSIGNMENT 3

Observation
1. Define what behaviour or behaviours you are going to observe.
2. Outline the method you are going to use either as a team or individually. Draw up the necessary recording forms and state the information you hope to observe.
3. Record observations and graph results. Set a baseline period of 5, 10, 15 days, etc., for your observations.
4. Present results and lead a group discussion with the support of your supervisors.

ASSIGNMENT 4

Observation
1. Pair up with a student, colleague, parent, or supervisor.
2. Set 5 minutes each to observe each other doing a task.
3. Record your observations of each other's behaviour during this period.
4. Discuss recordings with each other and supervisor or team members.
5. Now your supervisor/tutor and other team members should observe and record their observations of one mentally handicapped child. (Select a particular behaviour in advance.)
6. Check the amount of agreement/disagreement between observers.
7. Repeat this exercise for various behaviours reducing the amount of time for observation, e.g. 5 minutes, 4 minutes, 2 minutes, 1 minute.

8. Aim to 'sharpen' your observations and accurately record them during the reduction of time for observation periods. Also attempt to record relevant observations — that is the behaviours selected for the exercise. Recording of irrelevant behaviour, if made, should be openly discussed with tutors and in each team.

Note: Identification and discussion of irrelevant observations often proves helpful in training. It is important to know the pitfalls of observations, e.g. irrelevant recorded observations may lead to ineffective and inappropriate therapy plans and therefore poor therapeutic practice.

5

The therapy plan

PLANNING THERAPY

Planning therapy involves deciding what new behaviour mentally handicapped children are to learn and how they are going to achieve it. Sound therapy planning leads to successful therapy and job satisfaction for the therapist.

When an accurate personal assessment profile has been established, the nurse should then work with parents, a clinical psychologist, and other relevant team personnel to plan therapy for each individual. The discussion of *what* behaviours should be learnt in therapy should always include the *way* in which the behaviours are going to be taught. Sometimes the nurse will have to plan to reduce or extinguish 'bad habits'.* On other occasions, therapy will be planned to promote new behaviours, e.g. sharing, feeding, dressing, and carrying out domestic skills like cooking simple meals. Whatever behaviours are to be planned for therapy they should aim to fulfil the child's needs. In the past there have sadly been cases where, for instance, the needs of nursing personnel have been met at the cost of those of the mentally handicapped. This view is perhaps more true of mentally handicapped children living in long-stay hospitals. Whenever possible mentally handicapped children should have the opportunity of staying with their parents or in some place like home. Planning therapy in the interest of mentally handicapped children, their parents, and other caregivers should be considered under at least three categories.

Basic categories for planning therapy

1. *Reduction category*. Find out what behaviour or behaviours it is that have to be reduced or extinguished.

---

* As a general principle, when therapy is planned to reduce problem behaviour (bad habits), consideration should also be given to what alternative behaviours should be learned and increased during therapy.

2. *Promotion category.* Identify and define the behaviours the child needs to develop and maintain.
3. *Therapy steps.* Decide *how much* behaviour the child should learn in any one therapy session (this will often mean breaking down behaviours into 'bits' of behaviour that the child can learn successfully during each therapy session).

As I have said earlier, therapy should always start and end with success for the mentally handicapped child. Beginning and ending with success is rewarding both to the child and to the nurse. Success encourages the child and the nurse to try harder during therapy sessions. Such success often reinforces behaviours which have been learnt in therapy. When this happens it is likely that the behaviours which have been reinforced will occur more often. Reinforcement is a major part of therapeutic nursing and is considered in greater detail in the next chapter.

When the categories for carrying out therapy have been identified, the next step can be tackled by the nurse. This should be done in two stages:

(1) defining the target behaviour (the behaviour to be learnt);
(2) analysing the target behaviour (the size of the steps or 'bits' of behaviour to be learnt).

DEFINING TARGETS

Defining targets for therapeutic management means helping the child to learn the behaviours that have been chosen as targets for therapy. There are short-term and long-term goals in target behaviours. For example, a short-term goal might be to achieve the target of being able to get dressed without help. A long-term goal might be dressing, undressing, self-feeding, not being destructive, sharing toys with other children, etc. The type of target behaviours that the nurse should try to help the child to learn will depend largely on how quickly the child learns and how much is learnt during therapy sessions. The target behaviours for therapy will also be largely influenced by other factors, such as the skill of the nurse, the degree of involvement by parents, and the present level of the child's abilities. The range of behaviours already expressed should be assessed in order to identify the target behaviours the child should learn during therapy.

Using the developmental scales is a useful general approach to identifying target behaviours. Each child will have their own developmental profile of abilities. This will usually be reflected in the baseline period assessment. Enthusiastic nurses might feel they would like to avoid baseline period assessments and select a wide range of therapy targets for say, dressing, feeding, and toiletting. This may be possible for some children but tasks should usually be learned separately. This is with the intention of ensuring success and reward during therapy for the child. Alternatively, when combining therapy targets nurses should take into account the way in which they may be brought together. For instance, dressing and undressing are closely linked to toiletting. However, a more complex therapy plan might include intake of food — feeding — with toiletting — taking down pants, wiping, and pulling pants up. It is usually advisable and helpful to select target behaviours separately for the child, then string them together so that the same complex repertoire of feeding, dressing, and toiletting behaviour is achieved.

There are a number of different techniques which can be used in combination with reinforcement and punishment. These are discussed in greater detail when we consider therapeutic techniques. It must be stressed again, however, that the detailed and comprehensive assessment and identification of target behaviours for therapy must take place before therapy begins.

ANALYSING TARGET BEHAVIOUR

Analysing target behaviours for therapy involves breaking down the behaviour to be learnt into different steps which can each be achieved in one therapy session. In practice, this often means dividing a skill (e.g. washing, dressing, toiletting, feeding, etc.), into bits of behaviour which, when combined in an orderly sequence, make up the target behaviour. Selecting targets and analysing target behaviours for therapy are absolutely essential for valid therapy planning and success. The aim of all therapy should be to help the mentally handicapped to help themselves and become independent of their appointed therapists such as parents, nurses, and psychologists.

Here is a typical example of defining target behaviour and analysing it for the practice of therapeutic management.

Jane is severely mentally handicapped. She is 12 years old, knows parts of her body and can name them and point to them on verbal request. She usually demonstrates co-operative behaviour towards adults and does not express any 'problem behaviours'. Jane is also toilet-trained and eats without fuss or mess. She uses a spoon, but not a knife or fork. In dressing, she can take off all her clothes, but cannot put them all on yet. She carries out and understands simple instructions related to daily living. When she speaks, she uses one-word and occasionally two-word combinations. She does not wash or dry her hands.

When a personal assessment profile like this is derived from baseline observations, it is often appropriate to identify a single target behaviour for therapy. The team of therapists likely to be involved with Jane — parents, nursing personnel, and psychologists — would then meet, discuss, and agree upon a target behaviour they wanted Jane to learn, and how it was to be taught during therapeutic practice.

Let us say the therapeutic management team decided it was in Jane's interest for her to learn to wash and dry her hands. In doing this, they have identified the target behaviour for therapy. The behaviour has then to be analysed and divided into different seqential steps where Jane can gain early success, recognition, and reward for her achievement, for each of the behaviours involved in the target behaviour washing and drying hands. One approach to analysing and dividing the present therapy target can be detailed in the way shown in Table 5.1.

TABLE 5.1

Therapy target — washing and drying hands

Therapy steps

1. Walk to wash-basin.	9. Rub hands together.
2. Put plug in wash-basin.	10. Rinse hands in water.
3. Turn on tap.	11. Pull out plug.
4. Turn off tap.	12. Pick up towel.
5. Pick up soap.	13. Dry hands on towel.
6. Wet hands in water.	14. Replace towel.
7. Rub soap on hands.	15. Move away from wash-basin.
8. Put down soap.	

Each of these behaviours can be taught independently, increasing the number until the target behaviour has been achieved. Alternatively, larger 'chunks' of behaviour may be taught during therapy sessions. Exceptionally, all of the behaviour could be modelled (demonstrated) by the nurse and the child then encouraged and rewarded for imitating as much of the target behaviour as possible. Making the target behaviour more likely to occur should be one of the main concerns of the nurse. When target behaviour occurs, it should be reinforced. Reinforcement makes the behaviour which has taken place more likely to occur again. In this sense, all therapy should be concerned with the reinforcement of target behaviours. Reinforcement is explained in detail in the next chapter.

REMINDER

To achieve successful target behaviours, it is essential to pursue a genuine team approach towards therapy. This should be carried out comprehensively during the baseline period assessment and the therapy planning stages of therapeutic management. Working together, psychologists, parents, nurses, social workers, teachers, and other relevant personnel, should identify suitable and agreed ways of economically achieving therapy targets.

ASSIGNMENT 5

Therapy targets

1. Each member of the training team should discuss what therapy targets they are going to select for a therapy plan, with a particular mentally handicapped child.
2. The therapy targets should be expressed clearly and discussed with the tutor, parents, and mentally handicapped child (if this is possible). The discussion should centre around including one or more therapy targets into a therapy plan which may be put into practice.
3. Draw up therapy targets for therapy plan and decide which therapy planning categories they fall into.
4. Present the different stages of the assignment, and any difficulties which occur with your tutor/supervisor. Discuss the implications of the assignment — particularly with reference as to how it may or may not help to meet the needs of the handicapped person the individual team has chosen to work with.

ASSIGNMENT 6

1. Without reference to team members, individuals should carry out the above assignment.
2. Comparison of both approaches — team and individual, should then be made with tutors/supervisors and members of your own team.

6

Reinforcement and punishment

WHAT IS REINFORCEMENT?

This is a question which is not asked nearly often enough by behaviour therapists, perhaps because it is thought to be generally understood. However, for the purposes of behaviour therapy it should be made clear how it is used throughout this book. The definition of reinforcement used here is 'the stressing of a relationship between a response (behaviour) and consequences which follow it, so as to increase the probability of that response (behaviour)'.

This means that reinforcement increases the likelihood of the behaviour it follows. Therefore reinforcement of behaviour is concerned with increasing behaviour of any particular kind. So when we talk of *positive reinforcement* during therapy with mentally handicapped children we mean increasing desired behaviour by giving 'rewards' of one kind or another. Similarly when we talk of *negative reinforcement* (this is where there is often misunderstanding) it means increasing desired behaviour by removing 'penalties' of one kind or another.

By contrast 'punishment' is defined as any event which is contingent (dependent upon) an undesired behaviour, and which helps to reduce it. Punishment is therefore concerned with reducing undesirable behaviour and is *not* to be confused with negative reinforcement.

AN EXAMPLE OF REINFORCEMENT AND PUNISHMENT

Applying reinforcement and punishment to our own experience can give us some idea of how important the role reinforcement plays in behaviour therapy. Suppose we wanted to increase smiling behaviour in a friend. We could give them a pound note every time they smiled. The result would probably be an increase in smiling. In an instance like this we can say that they pound note reinforced smiling behaviour.

Now suppose we wanted to decrease smiling behaviour. The opposite procedure would be adopted. Each time the person smiled we would immediately take a pound away from them. The result would probably be a decrease in smiling behaviour (and possibly some demand for the return of the money we have taken).

In this example the pound note acts both as reinforcement and punishment of smiling behaviour. Notice that it is essential to administer or remove reinforcement and punishment immediately after a specified behaviour occurs, for they play a major part in therapeutic practice — in particular the use of reinforcement. There are at least three categories that have to be considered before proceeding with behaviour therapy.

1. When a child maintains or increases a particular way of behaving as a consequence of something consistently occurring which they like, we describe this as *reinforcement*.
2. When a child stops behaving in a particular way as a consequence of something consistently occurring which they dislike, we describe this as *punishment*.
3. When a child behaves in a particular way and we are unable to identify the consequences as ones which they like or dislike we cannot say whether reinforcement or punishment has occurred.

Clearly it is imperative to know what acts as reinforcement and punishment of behaviour for each individual child.

THE ROLE OF REWARDS IN REINFORCEMENT

Usually a wide range of rewards are used for reinforcement. The nurse will often want to reinforce desirable behaviours, such as social behaviours or skills related to the self-help. To do this effectively, personalized rewards must be identified for each child (the personal reward profile should be used here, see p.116). Reinforcement is often overlooked in planning therapy, and in particular in practising it. For instance, inappropriately selected rewards may even act as punishment for behaviour we actually want the child to learn, e.g. using ice-cream as a reward to reinforce behaviour when, in fact, the child detests the stuff! *Always have a systematic strategy for selecting appropriate rewards to be used in the potential reinforcement of behaviour.*

There are three practical ways to identify rewards to be used in positive reinforcement of behaviour during therapy:

1. Try out a wide range of rewards to see which one, or which combinations the child 'likes' best.
2. Identify rewards for positive reinforcement of behaviour from the child's past behaviour. In other words, try to identify aspects of the reinforcement history of each child, e.g. discussion with parents, past records, etc.
3. Identify personal rewards to use as positive reinforcement from the child's present behaviour. Baseline period observations should be used in such an instance.

There are 'primary reinforcers' and 'secondary reinforcers' which may act either as rewards or penalties when using them in therapy programmes. Many children cannot tell us when they do not like a 'reward' which has been chosen for them. Therefore, there is all the more reason for careful scrutiny of rewards for reinforcement of behaviour. Additionally, primary reinforcers and secondary reinforcers are a misnomer, until they have actually demonstrated reinforcement of any specified behaviour. In fact, we should really call them primary rewards, and secondary rewards, until reinforcement of behaviour occurs. It is at that moment the rewards takes on the effect of a reinforcer. Keeping this distinction in mind, it is possible to give a short list of typical primary and secondary rewards which have been used as effective reinforcers of behaviour with normal and mentally handicapped people.

PRIMARY REWARDS:

Edible: little sweets, chocolate, small sips of soft drinks, ice cream, nuts, raisins, popcorn, small pieces of fruit, cheese, vegetables, bread, etc.

SECONDARY REWARDS:

Movement and play: football, climbing, painting, playing with rocking-horse, simple games such as run-and-catch, hide-and-seek, etc.
Social rewards: kisses, hugs, stroking, smiling, praise, applause, etc.
Token rewards: these are usually discs which can be exchanged for something tangible, e.g. edible rewards. May also be exchanged for real money.

Reminder

It is prudent practice to clearly identify the rewards to be used as potential reinforcers during therapy.

There are also a number of general practical guidelines to adopt when practising therapy with the mentally handicapped child. These may be regarded as vital 'do's' and 'don'ts' of reward in therapeutic practice.

SOME DO'S AND DON'TS OF REWARDING MENTALLY HANDICAPPED CHILDREN

Do reward the child *immediately* the response you are looking for occurs. This avoids rewarding a behaviour that is not planned in the therapy. It also precludes the possibility of rewarding undesirable behaviour. On the positive side, it clearly conveys to the child which behaviours are being rewarded and which are not. Reinforcement of behaviour is likely to occur under these therapy conditions.

Do be *clear* and *enthusiastic* when you reward a child or adolescent for a specified behaviour. The child should be made aware by the therapist what behaviour it is that is being rewarded.

Do reward a child for desired behaviour or new skills *frequently*. To begin with the child needs to be rewarded every time the behaviour planned for therapy occurs. Later, when the desired response not only appears, but is established, rewards need not be used to reinforce behaviours so often.

Do make a careful and systematic assessment of the kinds of rewards to be used. *Reward selection* should aim to show what range of rewards to use, e.g. primary — edible — followed by secondary — social praise, etc. The targets for therapy should also influence the rewards to be used as potential reinforcers of behaviour. For instance, it is more effective and valid to use food as a reward in a feeding programme than social praise. Such rewards would also tend to 'naturally' maintain the behaviour they reinforce.

Don't *over-use rewards*. Mentally handicapped children, like their normal contemporaries, may become uninterested, bored, or habituated to 'reward saturation'. Typical signs of this can be seen in low co-operative behaviour in therapy, withdrawal from contact with the nurse, and occasionally assertive behaviour. These assertive behaviours need not necessarily be 'problem' behaviours. For instance, pushing, covering up the eyes, throwing the nurse's recording sheets away, or tearing them up can be 'healthy' indications of adolescent development. In such cases, the nurse should be prepared to alter the course of therapy, but *first* and *always* these observations should be discussed with other members of the therapeutic team. Communication of difficulties should not be seen as a failure, rather, as part of the process of adapting therapy to the needs of the mentally handicapped child. Communication and cross-consultation with parents, colleagues, and other professions, such as psychologists, should become established as standard procedure and reflected in therapeutic practice.

Reminder

Don't assume that the same rewards act as positive reinforcers for every mentally handicapped child (perhaps one of the most common mistakes that nurses and other therapists make). It is true that many rewards, e.g. fruit, chocolate, patting, stroking, are liked by many children, but *all* children do not like the same things. This *includes* the mentally handicapped child. Remember to *fit rewards to the individual's needs*. A reward to one child may be a punishing experience to others.

Do show that edible and movement rewards are associated with social rewards. This should be conveyed in your everyday contact with the mentally handicapped child. But avoid confusing the child by clearly *ordering* the way in which rewards of different kinds are to be given during therapy. Otherwise, it is difficult — almost impossible — to identify which rewards have reinforced the target behaviours identified for therapy.

Finally, **do** aim to reward behaviour which has been generalized by the child. This means rewarding behaviour which you wish to see transferred from one situation to another, e.g. urinating appropriately in different toilets, appropriate dining behaviour in different snack-bars, restaurants, and at home. Although rewards should be used in reinforcement of behaviour whenever possible, it will also be necessary to employ penalties in the presence of certain behaviour. This area of therapy is concerned with punishment.

PUNISHMENT

Like reinforcement, punishment has often been misunderstood. Punishment is often taken as a synonym for cruelty — this is not so in the way we use the term here. Certainly there are some kinds of therapy that involve corporal punishment, for example, electric shock therapy which may be necessary as a last resort to reduce or extinguish apparently intractable problem behaviours such as self-injury (Zangwill 1980). This is only one form of penalty-giving in nursing therapy. But there are a number of others that may be considered for therapeutic practice. These involve employing and removing penalties, and using words which may act as punishment or reinforcement during therapy.

Penalties and punishment

Corporal penalties. The most common notion of 'punishment' is using corporal penalties. Certain sorts of behaviour such as hyper-activity, pica, and the forms of self-injury found in Lesch-Nyham's syndrome can be punished with for instance, a smack on the hand or a spank on the seat. This form of penalty is often difficult to justify on practical, therapeutic, and ethical grounds. Corporal penalties should not, as a general rule, be used in order to reduce undesirable behaviour. From a practical point of view, they have only short-term deterrent effects upon undesirable behaviour. Additionally, it may act as a model of behaviour for the mentally handicapped child to adopt in their interactions with other people. The therapeutic pay-off from using corporal penalties is, therefore, of short-term benefit, in contrast to the cost-effect it may have on other behaviours of the mentally handicapped. Taking practical, professional, and ethical arguments into consideration, other alternatives are more attractive and suitable.

Alternative to corporal penalties

1. *Application and removal of penalties.* When undesirable behaviour occurs penalties are imposed. But after a period of its absence, it is important to remove penalties that may have been imposed, e.g. terminating threats; stopping scolding or shouting; allowing the child to return to sit with the rest of the class or to join in the family dinner, and so on. This is a constructive use of punishment quickly followed by negative reinforcement.
2. *Removal of rewards.* Removing rewards can be used for undesirable behaviour. This should be done immediately after the behaviour has occurred. Switching off the TV, stopping smiling, not allowing the child to talk, not allowing him to have a bicycle ride, terminating your walk with him, turning off music, etc., are a few examples.

---

* The clinical manifestations of pica are the ingestion of inedible substances, such as paint, wood, etc. It occurs in children throughout all levels of intelligence. However, the behaviour seems to be more common amongst the mentally handicapped population.

Extinction

This is another way in which rewards can be removed. Extinction is the active and controlled employment of non-reward. This is a penalty which is not always easily implemented in therapy. It requires great discipline on the behalf of the therapist. Examples of extinction in practice involves ignoring predetermined selected responses that are made by the child, e.g. ignoring the child who shouts instead of talking to him or playing with him. Many behaviours fail to become extinguished in the mentally handicapped child at home, school, or in the hospital, largely because they continue to be reinforced by parents, teachers, and nursing personnel who 'mean well'. In other words, we often reward and maintain the very behaviours which we would like to see disappear. When a specific behaviour no longer occurs, or is emitted at a very low rate, it is said to be extinguished.

A complication in the use of extinction is the appearance of an apparent 'worsening' of problem behaviours. An increase in the rate, frequency, and duration of problem behaviour may become evident. This can be seen as a resistance effect, which then eventually reduces and becomes extinguished. The error to avoid here is giving up practising the therapy or prejudging therapy as a failure because of an increase in problem behaviour is observed and recorded.

One final word about extinction, it is usually sound practice to combine extinction with the reinforcement of alternative desirable behaviours. In the example above, the child who shouts should be rewarded for asking or speaking in a lower voice. Rewarding of this alternative desirable behaviour, if successful, will reinforce acceptable voice behaviour — something which is in the interests of the mentally handicapped child, the parents, peers, teachers, and whoever else comes into contact with the child. Using extinction on its own, has often led to so-called 'symptom substitution'. For instance, solely and actively ignoring shouting might effectively extinguish shouting, but be replaced by headbanging or some other form of self-injurious behaviour. Symptom substitution is not, however, typical. Another practice which has produced effective therapeutic results is called 'time-out training'.

TIME-OUT TRAINING

Employing time-out training in therapeutic nursing must be done after the closest consideration of all the possible ways in which the child can be helped to acquire or decrease specified behaviours. The team of therapists involved in any particular therapy employing time-out procedures should be satisfied that it is going to be used in the interest of the child.

Time-out training involves using both removal of rewards and imposing penalties — in that order. In time-out the child may be taken away from a rewarding-reinforcing situation, or the source of the reward-reinforcement taken away from them. In either case a penalty is being imposed by the nurse for behaviour which has to be punished. For example, a child who does not wait their turn to have their morning fruit-juice and who engages in temper tantrums, is either taken away from the juice or the juice is removed from the table unit until the tantrum has subsided. At this point the penalty is then removed — the child is taken back to the table where the juice is, or the juice is brought back to the table for the child to drink. It must be emphasized that time-out training should concern itself with rewarding as well as the punitive aspect of therapy. Lifting the penalty imposed by time-out when desired behaviours occur should be swiftly followed through with reward-reinforcement of skill-building and socially acceptable behaviours.

When time-out training is adopted by nurses, they should carefully consider and discuss with parents, their colleagues, and psychologists the length of time a penalty is to be employed, for instance, if 30 seconds away from a reward-reinforcement situation or more is to be practised in therapy. As a general guideline, it is unhelpful, as well as unethical, to impose time-out penalties for long periods — say more than five minutes — during therapy. Moreover, from the purely practical point of view, employing prolonged penalties can have the effect of punishing behaviour which was not a target for therapy, e.g. sitting quietly in a case where the therapy target is sitting behaviour. Penalties should only be used to maximize therapeutic effect. In practice this means achieving targets without infringing the rights of the mentally handicapped or underestimating their needs.

ASSIGNMENT 7

Reinforcement and punishment

1. Outline with team colleagues what is meant by reinforcement and punishment.

2. Identify someone you have been working with and report the way in which reinforcement or punishment may be employed therapeutically to promote their further development.
3. Discuss the practical and ethical issues surrounding the notion of punishment.
4. Keep notes of this assignment to raise in future during occasions when there is a need to clarify the similarities and differences between reinforcement and punishment.
5. Present a summary of the assignment to your tutor/supervisor for further group discussion and individual assessment.

Methods of reinforcement

SCHEDULES OF REINFORCEMENT

Various methods of reinforcement are used by psychologists to encourage the behavioural development of the mentally handicapped. These are usually referred to as 'schedules of reinforcement', and are also used in nursing therapy. The three main methods used in nursing therapy are continuous reinforcement, interval reinforcement, and ratio reinforcement. Knowing which of these categories they are using will help nurses to evaluate their programmes of therapy.

CONTINUOUS REINFORCEMENT

Recall that we may practise positive or negative inforcement. Continuous reinforcement simply refers to maintaining or increasing a desired form of behaviour by always following it with a reward or the removal of a penalty. For instance, when we observe somebody feeding themselves we see that they are behaving under a schedule of continuous positive reinforcement. Every time the person places a spoonful of food in their mouth (behaviour) the food (reward) has the effect (reinforcement) or maintaining feeding behaviour. When the food is finished, or the individual pushes the remaining food away, it has ceased to have a reward value for them; it no longer has the effect of reinforcement. Similarly, should we observe the person actively seeking more food, this would show that stopping the continuous presentation of a food reward results in an increase of food-seeking behaviour. In such a case, the increase in behaviour can be seen as the individual's attempt to obtain reinforcement.

Another typical example of continuous positive reinforcement is when the nurse presents a primary or secondary reward, such as chocolate or praise, every time the child looks at the nurse, picks up a toy, says 'please', rubs wet hair with towel, and other instances where a reward is always presented immediately *after* a behaviour to be reinforced. When nurses use this method they are practising a schedule of continuous positive reinforcement.

One example of continuous negative reinforcement often used by nurses is scolding the child until he stops running away from the medication area. Less obvious however is the mentally handicapped child who continuously negatively reinforces the nurse. For example, the child who stops shouting when the nurse tries to calm him 'down'. Mistakenly, it is often thought that the calming down works. But on further analysis it is revealed the nurse's behaviour is operating on a schedule of continuous negative reinforcement carried out by the child. Looking at this another way, the child shouts or screams until the nurse attempts to reduce the shouting. But in terms of reinforcement, the child has used undesirable behaviour to *increase* the approach and interaction from the nurse. Some children may even be prepared to injure themselves in order to receive the involvement of their parents or nurse. Simply, the child who engages in anti-social behaviour or self-injury may in many cases have learnt that it is one of the few ways to obtain rewards from this environment. Similarly, the nurse may have learnt to wait for the unacceptable behaviour before moving in to help the child. When this has happened an insidious transaction between the nurse and the child will have been established on the principle of continuous negative reinforcement. It is imperative that this sort of interpersonal behaviour is changed — even though it may mean some short-term acute anxiety experienced by the nurse. Ignoring this problem when it arises will not facilitate its reduction, but only serve to maintain the 'problem' behaviour.

INTERVAL REINFORCEMENT

Interval reinforcement is a method which relies on presenting rewards or removing penalties *after* a predetermined period of *time* has elapsed on the occasion of a specified behaviour's being present. When practising interval reinforcement nurses should be clear whether they are using what has been termed *fixed* interval reinforcement or *variable* interval reinforcement. Fixed interval reinforcement is used to reward a child after a set period of time in order to reinforce specified behaviour. For instance, it might be agreed by the nurse and the therapeutic team that 'Eric' should be rewarded to reinforce sharing behaviour with other children. If Eric is placed in a play situation for 30 minutes, it might be decided to set a fixed interval period of praise (secondary reward) at the end of every five-minute period for the entire play session. In this case, Eric would be rewarded with praise during his play to reinforce sharing behaviour, using a *fixed interval* positive reinforcement schedule of five minutes. The point about fixed interval reinforcement is that it is administered by the nurse at the end of the same period of time throughout the entire schedule of reinforcement. However, the nurse may want to change the fixed interval to an interval reinforcement schedule of every 10 minutes. In Eric's case, if the play session was still 30 minutes long, he would be rewarded on three occasions on a 10-minute fixed interval schedule of reinforcement.

Where the nurse and the therapeutic team decided to reward Eric first after 5, then 10, then 15 minutes this would be adopting a *variable interval* schedule of positive reinforcement. In variable interval schedules of reinforcement, the nurse should practise presenting rewards or removing penalties after the predetermined interval period has been reached. For instance, if a 5-1-15-10-minute variable interval schedule of reinforcement was to be practised during therapy, the nurse would present or remove penalties immediately at the ends of these interval periods. So, if 'Rose' is to be rewarded to achieve reinforcement for temper-tantrum-free periods, the nurse might adopt a variable interval schedule or positive reinforcement similar to the above. Let us say that temper-tantrum-free episodes were rewarded using the 5-1-15-10-minute variable interval schedule of reinforcement. The aim of this schedule of positive reinforcement would be to promote and expand the periods of time where temper tantrums did not occur. Both the fixed interval and variable interval schedules of reinforcement are essentially concerned with increasing the amount of *time* specified tantrum-free behaviour can be maintained or increased. The important difference between fixed and variable interval reinforcement which the nurse should remember from the mentally handicapped child's viewpoint, is their degree of predictability. Where children are receiving a fixed-interval schedule of reinforcement, they may learn to predict when they will be rewarded or penalties removed for behaviour which is reinforced. By contrast, employing a variable-interval schedule of reinforcement, mentally handicapped children, like their normal peers, should learn that they are unlikely to predict when rewards will be presented to reinforce behaviour.

It is important to recognize these distinctions. If we continue the example of 'Eric' and 'Rose' we can see why Eric was rewarded to achieve reinforcement of sharing behaviour on a fixed interval schedule of positive reinforcement, whereas a variable schedule of positive reinforcement was practised with 'Rose'.

In the fixed interval schedule Eric learned to predict that he could be rewarded for sharing. In this case a specific level of his play behaviour was reinforced. It may also have been appropriate to use a variable interval schedule of reinforcement with him. However, it would not have been clear to him why he was being rewarded and what behaviour was being reinforced. For Rose, it seemed appropriate to use a variable interval schedule of positive reinforcement for temper-tantrum-free episodes because the nurse wanted her to learn that reward came during different periods but not to predict *when* they would be presented by the therapist. The reasoning behind this schedule was to avoid a situation where Rose learnt to provide temper-tantrum-free behaviour only on the periods immediately prior to a reward being presented. These particular cases serve to illustrate two general points for nurses. First, where the therapist wishes to maintain or expand behaviour which is already present, fixed interval schedules of reinforcement should be used. It is also likely that variable interval schedules of reinforcement will probably also work in situations of this sort. Second, where the therapist wants the child to learn to predict the consequences of their behaviour they should adopt fixed rather than variable interval schedules of reinforcement in therapeutic procedure.

RATIO REINFORCEMENT

Ratio reinforcement refers to the methods which rely on presenting rewards or removing penalties immediately after a specific *number* of occasions a specified behaviour occurs. Like interval reinforcement, ratio reinforcement may be practised by *fixed or variable ratio* schedules of reinforcement.

Fixed ratio reinforcement is practised by counting a constant number of behaviours before presenting rewards or removing penalties. Immediately the set number of behaviours have occurred the nurse should present the reward or remove the penalty. A typical example of fixed ratio positive reinforcement can be seen in the case of sorting tasks. Sorting is essentially concerned with grouping classes of items together. The task might be to sort different items into groups or to sort out particular items from a larger group. Fixed ratio positive reinforcement can be applied to these tasks in play or training in work skills. How would the nurse proceed with reinforcing sorting behaviour? First the nurse would identify the nature of the sorting task. If it were sorting groups of metal tags from plastic ones, the nurse's task might be to give reinforcement for all correctly sorted metal tags. So no reinforcement would be given for incorrect sorting. But fixed ratio reinforcement would be used when the task was to sort metal tags into separate groups, say, sets of six. Here the nurse would only present the reward after the correct sixth metal tag was selected into the group. This example demonstrates a number of further points which are common to fixed ratio reinforcement and reinforcement in general.

First, before any schedule of reinforcement is practised, the task which the nurse wishes the child to learn should be clearly identified. Secondly, once this has been done, it is prudent practice to check what parts of the task the child can already perform, and those yet to be learnt. For instance, if in the sorting task example above, a child could not yet sort metal tags from plastic ones, there would be no point in proceeding to practise rewarding after every sixth tag had been selected. In this event, reinforcement might lead to the child's learning that any selection of six tags would be rewarded. The underlying message here to nurses is clear. Not only should the kind of task be clearly identified and how much of it the person can do — but equal attention should be paid to how and in what way the therapist reinforces the behaviour to be learnt. This is a principle of all schedules of reinforcement.

Variable ratio reinforcement is closely connected to fixed ratio reinforcement. The difference lies in the number of times a behaviour occurs before reinforcement is practised. Whereas the fixed ratio schedule relies on a set number, variable ratio reinforcement is employed by variations in the number of times a behaviour occurs immediately before behaviour reinforcement is practised.

Desirable social behaviour, is a wide area where variable ratio schedules of reinforcement can be practised. Dining table courtesy which entails sitting at a table with others, sharing bread, passing cutlery, handling crockery, and taking turns at serving food, can all be linked to *variable ratio* schedules of reinforcement using secondary social rewards. Where a child has difficulty in any of these behaviours and when some appropriate change has been indicated (for example by continuous positive reinforcement) the nurse may move on to variable ratio reinforcement. In such a case the nurse may decide to practise reinforcement after the 1st, 2nd, 5th, 8th, 9th, 14th, and 20th meal of each week. Echoing the practice of variable interval reinforcement the nurse could continue appropriate dining table courtesy on the predetermined days for ratio reinforcement. In other words selected secondary rewards such as praise, smiling, patting, and talking to the child would be practised on the 1st, 2nd, 5th, 8th, 9th, 14th, and 20th meals of each week. Two points should be noted here: first, it is not an arbitrary therapeutic practice; and secondly variable ratio reinforcement may be effectively practised *after* a person's behaviour has become established under some other schedule of reinforcement. This seems to be the case for interval reinforcement also. Although there is no immutable rule for the practice of variable schedules of reinforcement, the nurse should first get experience with continuous reinforcement and fixed interval and ratio reinforcement before moving on to applying variable schedules of reinforcement. The main reason for this is that the nurse should attain control over the therapy being practised. In doing so, gaining control over the practice of continuous reinforcement, and fixed schedules of reinforcement should gradually lead to control over the practice of variable interval and fixed interval reinforcement. Achieving control over the practice of the different schedules of reinforcement is also a reflection of the nurse's level of therapeutic competence. The more nurses can control the practice of the schedule of reinforcement, the more they control the way they employ rewards and penalties. When control over the practice of the schedules of reinforcement has been obtained, the nurse should then be in a position to effectively combine them with the different therapy techniques presented in the following chapter.

ASSIGNMENT 8

1. Draw up a list of the various ways in which reinforcement might be practised by your therapy team.
2. Select a number of actual problems which a mentally handicapped child reflects in his behaviour and decide the most appropriate method of reinforcement for each problem.

3. Select a number of appropriate behaviours which should be maintained by the mentally handicapped children you know and decide on the most suitable method of reinforcement to maintain these behaviours.

4. Present your ideas of reinforcement methods and the reasons for selecting particular schedules of reinforcement to carry out behaviour therapy with the mentally handicapped. Use printed handouts and audio-visual aids to illustrate your assignment. Carry out this part of the assignment with the support of your tutor-supervisor.

8

Therapy techniques

ATTENTION

Before observable progress can be made it is essential to first engage the attention of the mentally handicapped child. Similarly, if normal children do not attend to tasks which they are expected to learn, e.g. spelling, reading, and arithmetic, their rate of learning on these tasks becomes impaired. Mentally handicapped children should, therefore, first 'pay attention' to the therapy targets they are to learn. If this basic attending behaviour is not first established, much of the therapy becomes a waste of time and effort. The first task in deciding which techniques to employ in therapy is to discover whether or not attending behaviour is present. There are three main reasons why attending behaviour should be present:

1. The child will have the opportunity of learning from the nurse faster than when attending behaviour is absent.
2. The child will have the opportunity of learning appropriate behaviours selected for therapy.
3. The child will have taken the first steps to being co-operative and participating in therapy.

What does attending behaviour involve? Does it merely mean looking at the therapist; listening to the therapist? Some combination of these two? Attending should involve at least looking and listening. If this is not possible (e.g. with the Rubella-affected child who has congenital deafness) the therapist must use the sensory channels available. However, in general, where the child does not suffer from deafness or blindness listening and looking are behaviours to look for in deciding whether or not the child is attending. This, in itself, is still not sufficient for carrying out effective therapy. Attending is an activity which, if it is to be applied to learning, must be selective (Lunzer 1970). It can be claimed that learning is based upon the application of selective attention and previous experience.

The child and the nurse make a sort of contract at the beginning of the therapy session. Usually the nurse will say the child's name followed by the command 'look at me'. So, for instance, if the nurse is trying to get a child to look at what she is doing she will say 'Mary, look at me'. This apparently simple approach is a checking technique to see if attending behaviour is present. It involves directed complicated selective attending on behalf of the child.

TABLE 8.1

An example of behavioural requirements for selective attending

Nurse	Child
Looks at child and selects name and command. (Expresses name and command. Uses tone appropriate to the command. Waits for response. Looks at child.)	Looks towards nurse on hearing own name. Responds to command as a result of the message 'Mary, look at me'. Ignores other extraneous stimulation.

These behavioural requirements are listed in Table 8.1 to demonstrate the intricate interaction and selective attending which takes place in establishing attending behaviour. For many children attending behaviour is maintained only for short periods of time, e.g. 10 seconds, 1 minute, 3 minutes, and so on. The point here is to decide if the attending behaviour that is present is adequate for the therapy to be employed. In other words, attending behaviour should be related to the duration and frequency of therapy sessions. In each case it should be decided whether or not sufficient, and therefore adequate, attending behaviour has been established before employing any therapy plan. If it is not, the therapy plan would then have to be revised to adopt attending behaviour as the primary therapy target.

'Shaping up' attending behaviour usually begins with the child's learning to look at the nurse or task to be learnt. The former behaviour is often referred to as obtaining 'eye-contact'. Two related techniques for promoting attending behaviour can be used: reward presentation and fading out.

Reward presentation

Reward presentation is important when therapy is aimed at getting the child's attention. The timing of the rewards presented to reinforce attending behaviour should correspond closely to the definition of attending behaviour which is to be reinforced. In other words, defining precisely what counts at an attending response must be done at the therapy planning stage. The team of therapists should be in no doubt what behaviour counts as attending. As a result, rewards can be presented consistently for different degrees of attending behaviour. For instance, it may be decided that 'John' should be rewarded for brief glances at the nurse or what he is doing. To begin with, these glances may only be of a few seconds' duration. This would have to be specified in advance of therapy, so that in actual practice John is rewarded for brief attending behaviour. Later he could be rewarded for longer periods of attending behaviour to the nurse or a task. One way of doing this would be to delay the reward given for the attending response. Alternatively, increased reward presentation could be practised for increasing the number of times Mary attended to the therapist or task she had to learn. At some point early on in the therapy, it should be established that 'John' or 'Mary' would start responding to their own names. The idea here is to get the children attending first to their own names (as we do) so that they will attend to a wide range of task behaviours. The aim of this approach is to help the child attend to communications like 'Mary, do this', 'Mary, watch me', 'Mary, look at me', 'Mary, what is this?', 'Mary, show me', etc. Using the first name a personalized approach should be encouraged as a routine practice amongst and between the nurses as well as their use of the child's name. The Johns and Marys of the mentally handicapped population need to have cues to attending to people and tasks. The most obvious form is using the personalized form of address. In addition to acting as a cue to attending behaviour, it recognizes the need the mentally handicapped child has in common with normal contemporaries — the need for individual recognition and a sense of personal identity.

Fading out

Sometimes it is necessary to achieve attention and response to personal address by a slightly different technique. This is often referred to as fading out. Here the idea is to gradually reduce the amount of reward for glancing and prolonged attending behaviour. This is something like delaying reward for eye-contact and attending. Attending behaviour is, therefore, increased over time.

Fading out, however also usually aims to remove the immediate reward for attending to a low level. For example, small pieces of fruit or nuts may be used to reward and reinforce a particular form of attending behaviour. When the attending behaviour has been established in sufficient strength, the sweets or nuts are gradually faded out. This can be done by presenting less of a reward, e.g. three sweets, two sweets, one sweet, etc. Where social approval of attending behaviour is employed as reward to reinforce attending behaviour, the frequency and duration of social approval can be decreased. For instance, complimenting the child for looking at the nurse or attending to work tasks could be reduced from 10 times per day and 15 seconds' duration on each occasion, to 3 times per day and 5 seconds' duration on each occasion. The level of fading out and the specific form it takes will depend upon the child and the attending behaviour required to be learnt. The nurse should also consider how to fade out unnecessary rewards and penalties, as well as rewarding the behaviours they want to maintain through reinforcement. In general a minimal level of reward has to be established in order to maintain attending behaviour. Using the personalized form of address and social approval with each child seems necessary to maintain attending behaviour. How often would we attend to someone who called us by someone else's name or never addressed us at all? Our own experience tells us 'very seldom', quickly leading to 'not at all'. In this example, extinction would have taken place and the aim of fading out lost. For, in fading out rewards, the nurse should aim to maintain the target behaviour set for therapy, whereas in extinction the nurse aims to reduce or eliminate behaviour.

When attending behaviour has been established, co-operation will also have begun to appear. The appearance of co-operative behaviour makes it possible to widen the range of targets to aim for during therapeutic practice.

CO-OPERATION

Once attending behaviour has been achieved, the nurse should then move on to helping the child to co-operate in the task of therapy. There are different aspects of co-operation, just as there are many intricacies of attending behaviour. In therapeutic nursing, the nurse is likely to be mainly concerned with three types of co-operation.

1. Co-operative behaviour which permits assessment to take place, e.g. sitting at a table, carrying out requests, trying harder, etc.
2. Co-operative behaviour which permits the child to engage in play or tasks which have been selected as target behaviours to learn in therapy. (It is often important to teach mentally handicapped children how to play, as well as showing them play things.)
3. Co-operative behaviour which permits the child to interact with his contemporaries, e.g. sharing toys, waiting turns, being one of a team making crafts, having good dining table 'manners', etc.

As with getting the attention of the child nurses will often have to 'shape up' the different kinds of co-operation required for any particular form of therapy. The three types of co-operation above are typical of the kinds of behaviour required for specific therapy tasks. However, they should not be used as recipes for therapeutic intervention. Rather, they should be seen as starting-points for building personal co-operation which will not obstruct further therapeutic practice.

Each child is different and therefore should be treated and respected as an individual. This means that the combination of establishing attending behaviour and co-operation will be a personal endeavour for each child. So, for instance, one child may only be able to attend and imitate what the nurse does, whereas another will attend and carry out complex verbal requests and initiate communication. When communication is initiated by the child, it is an important advance in the development of co-operation. Later, when we come to look at communicating we shall see that the nurse can use verbal and non-verbal techniques to assist the child to learn. This assistance in learning new behaviours involves using a number of other therapy techniques, such as shaping-chaining, prompting, integrating, and modelling.

SHAPING AND CHAINING

When we build up behaviours to help the mentally handicapped child to help themselves, shaping and chaining techniques are used.

These are particularly useful and practical for therapy which aims to establish play and independent skills in toiletting, dressing, and undressing. Self-catering skills can also be shaped up and chained together to produce different levels of independent behaviour — for instance making sandwiches and coffee.

Shaping and chaining involve behaviours which are built up gradually to produce a therapy target by moulding simple bits of behaviour into more complex forms, e.g. moving from looking at a spoon, to picking it up, to plunging it into food, to taking the spoon from the plate to the mouth, to opening the mouth and placing the spoon in the mouth, to removing the spoon from the mouth, to repeating the behaviour sequence known as 'feeding with a spoon'. Here, the feeding behaviours start at the simple level and gradually move to the more complex activity of feeding. Like many shaping techniques, the target behaviours, e.g. feeding, dressing, and undressing, are built up from units of behaviour (something which the nurse will work towards). The behaviours as they become more like the target behaviour, are said to achieve successive approximation. In other words, the 'best' successive approximation that can be made during therapy is reaching the target behaviour, e.g. the child's looking at you when you address them by name, showing you red 'means' stop and green 'means' go, selecting a 10 pence coin on request instead of a 2 pence or 5 pence one, etc. Often the nurse will have to use verbal prompts like 'yes', 'no', 'that's right', etc., as well as gestures and physical prompts like pointing or lightly physically guiding a correct response. Reward should often follow the behaviour, even though it has been prompted by the nurse.

Chaining behaviour together is not something which is a novel idea. Young infants do this when they are learning early self-care skills like feeding. Since reaching is necessary for feeding and knowing which part of the body the spoon has to travel towards, the infant has to practise reaching to build up feeding behaviour. The result is that normal infants move from being 'messy' to being 'clean' eaters. They learn to first move from low successive approximation to high successive approximation in feeding behaviour. To achieve this they also have to chain together the different units of behaviour that result in 'clean eater' status. The task is much the same for mentally handicapped children. They have to aim for high successive approximation to the target set for therapy and also connect all the units of behaviour together to produce, say, feeding.

In the example given so far each unit of chaining can be learnt in a forward sequence. This simply involves the child's learning the first part of a behaviour first and the last part at the end of the sequence. However, much of the behaviour promoting independence can also be learnt in reverse order. This is called backward chaining.

Backward chaining

Backward chaining aims therapy at learning the *last* unit of behaviour in the chain *first*. For example, in dressing if the child has to learn to dress himself, it involves being able to chain all of the behaviour associated with dressing. With this technique, putting on pants, shirt, trousers, sweater, socks, and shoes are learnt by rewarding and reinforcing learning of the behaviours in reverse order. A typical example of a dressing routine using this approach would be as shown in Table 8.2.

TABLE 8.2

Chain link	Instruction and behaviour learnt
1.	The child is completely dressed *except* for his shoes. The child's name is said for each instruction, followed by the words 'get dressed'. The child is immediately rewarded when he puts the shoes on (it may, of course, be necessary to help him with a physical prompt as well as verbal instruction).
2.	The child is dressed except for his shoes and socks. The therapist addresses the child by name and says 'David, get dressed' (again he is helped physically if necessary). He is immediately rewarded when he puts on the shoes and socks.
3.	The child is dressed except for sweater, socks, and shoes. Proceed as above.
4.	The child is dressed except for trousers, sweater, socks, and shoes. Proceed as above.
5.	The child is dressed except for shirt, trousers, sweater, sock and shoes. Proceed as above.
6.	The child is dressed except for pants, shirt, trousers, sweater, socks, and shoes. Proceed as above.
7.	The child is undressed. As before say 'David, get dressed'. David puts on pants, shirt, trousers, sweater, socks, and shoes. He can now dress himself.

The mentally handicapped child in this example has completed the task of dressing by backward chaining the dressing behaviour together. The end result: the target behaviour is complete independence in dressing. When nurses use this approach, they should also consider the *size* of steps to use as different links the child has to learn in the behaviour chain. Practise breaking down different behaviours in this way. It is a useful exercise to adopt prior to therapy practice. Analysing behaviour in this way is useful to the nurse in at least four ways:

1. It defines what is to be learnt during therapy.
2. It permits the nurse to decide when any part of the target behaviours in therapy have been achieved, e.g. how many steps in dressing or feeding have been learnt?
3. It makes it possible to decide the rate of learning for any particular individual using the size of the links in the behaviour chain to be learnt. In other words it is possible to discover how quickly the child learns the behaviours set for therapy.
4. It informs the therapist when to move on to new therapy targets.

Using this approach serves as another form of therapeutic strategy. Point one involves target definition — the answer to the question 'What is to be taught?'. Points 2 and 3 provide answers to the monitoring questions 'What has been learnt?' and 'How long has it taken to learn?' Point 4 answers the question 'What has to be learnt next?' These sound deceptively simple questions, but, in practice, it is necessary to find suitable methods of recording what has been learnt, how long it took to achieve target behaviours set for therapy, and what should be learnt in future. Discussing these issues with colleagues, parents, and all of the therapy team, should help to clarify how this sort of information might be observed, recorded, and monitored. Each therapy team should also design their own therapy recording forms. An example used for bladder and bowel training is shown below. It may not appeal to every team of therapists or even be suitable for every mentally handicapped child. However, it has proved helpful in providing answers to the questions raised above about therapeutic practice and the effectiveness of the techniques used.

BLADDER AND BOWEL BEHAVIOUR ANALYSIS (BABBA)

The bladder and bowel behaviour analysis (BABBA) consists of recording half-hourly condition of the child. Put the appropriate toiletting symbol in at each time check. So for instance, if the child is 'dry' at 8 a.m. enter D in the 8 a.m. box. Similarly if 'wet', 'soiled', 'urinated' (in toilet), or 'excreted' (defecated in toilet) mark in each capital letter at time check. Complete the BABBA chart in this way. At the end of the check period, you will have a profile of the child's bladder and bowel behaviour. Where the child shows two of the features such as being both wet *and* soiled at a time check, include in check box thus: WS. An example of how the chart has been used is given in Fig. 8.1. This example shows how valuable the BABBA chart is in identifying useful information to help the child. The record shows a baseline set of recordings over five days.

Points that the nurse should note are the pattern of bowel and bladder behaviour at check periods, and the overall profile to date. For instance, it is clear 'Anne' is not wet all of the time, nor is she soiled all of the time. It can be seen that at 10 a.m.-10.30 a.m. she urinates approximately in the toilet, and this is consistent to date. She is dry between 1 p.m. and 2.30 p.m. on the days she has been checked. This is also consistent. The overall profile suggests she is dry *most* of the time to date. Wetting is more frequent than soiling. There is a slight drop in her appropriate urinating but indications of an increase in defecating on the toilet.

Analysis of the BABBA chart could be pursued in greater detail and evaluated at any time during baseline assessments and during therapy. Two final points are worth making about this chart. First, it shows nurses that appropriate bladder and bowel behaviour is not totally absent. This should help the nurse to have a more accurate impression of the child's present learning pattern. Second, and related to this point, during baseline observations of this kind, the nurse may see an improvement in bladder and bowel behaviour as the checks progress. Again this seems to be evidence of the child's learning ability. Checking may act as a method for helping the child discriminate what has to be learnt. It also helps the nurse to avoid errors in pre-judging the effects of therapeutic practice.

Prompting

Shaping and chaining behaviour together is often helped by using various prompts. Using appropriate prompts helps the child to achieve target behaviours in therapy. There are physical, gestural, and verbal prompts:

Fig. 8.1.

Name: *Anne Elms*
Age: *14*
Date commenced recording: *1st August 1981*

Bladder and bowel behaviour analysis (BABBA)

Behaviour symbols: D = Dry S = Soiled W = Wet U = Urinated (in toilet) E = Excreted/defecated (in toilet)

Please record appropriate symbol each day and at each BABBA time check

Day	Initials of staff	A.M.														P.M.										Daily period BABBA				
		Half-hour time checks																													
		8/8½	8½/9	9/9½	9½/10	10/10½	10½/11	11/11½	11½/12	12/12½	12½/1	1/1½	1½/2	2/2½	2½/3	3/3½	3½/4	4/4½	4½/5	5/5½	5½/6	6/6½	6½/7	7/7½	7½/8	D	W	S	U	E
1	RB	W	D	D	ws	U	D	D	D	W	D	U	D	D	U	U	U	D	D	W	D	D	D	D	W	14	6	2	3	0
2	RB	W	D	D	D	D	D	D	D	W	W	D	D	S	W	U	D	D	U	W	D	D	W	W	W	15	5	1	3	0
3	AT	D	D	U	W	W	D	D	D	ws	D	U	D	S	U	D	D	D	U	D	D	W	D	D	S	14	5	2	3	0
4	·AT	W	S	D	D	D	D	D	W	W	D	S	D	S	S	D	D	D	W	D	D	E	D	D	D	15	4	3	1	1
5	AT	W	D	D	D	D	D	W	W	S	D	D	D	W	S	D	W	W	U	D	D	E	D	D	D	15	4	2	2	1
6																														
7																														
8																														
9																														
10																														
11																														
12																														
13																														
14																														
15																														
16																														
17																														
18																														
19																														
20																														
21																														
22																														
23																														
24																														
25																														
26																														
27																														
28																														
29																														
30																														
31																														
Total checks																														

Physical prompts. When physical prompts are used the child is bodily guided through each piece of behaviour by taking him 'through the motions'. So, if we were trying to get the child to pick something up we would take his hand and guide it with our own and pick up a spoon or a toy. In using physical prompts the nurse should aim to provide the maximum amount of help in carrying out an action. With physical prompts, the child *feels* through his own body and the action of his own hand what the nurse requires him to learn through the prompt. Sometimes physical prompts accompany or supplement gestural and verbal prompts.

Gestural prompts. When we get to the stage in therapy where physical prompts are no longer necessary, gestural prompts can be used. Gestural prompts are used to show the child what to do. This will often be the case after the nurse has established attention and co-operation. The use of gestural prompts is as important to children without hearing problems as they are for those who have difficulties in hearing and understanding what is said.

Using gestural prompts means simply and clearly showing the child what to do by mime. Using gesture alone, e.g. pointing, nodding or shaking the head, etc., the nurse shows the child what has to be learnt without touching him. The child then *sees* what to do in a gestural prompt. Gestural prompts are therefore used to communicate to children what is expected of them.

It is important that a child has adequate vision when gestural prompts are used. The child's eyesight should be checked before any therapy which uses gestural prompts is begun, since there is little use in trying to gesture to a child to tie his shoelaces if he cannot see the gesture clearly or, for that matter, the shoelaces.

Verbal prompts. With verbal prompts therapy is simply aimed at telling the child what we want him to do. Using this technique, the child *hears* what behaviour is expected of him by the nurse, e.g. 'Suzy, sit down', 'Eric, give me your plate', 'Peter, please take your orange juice'. The child with hearing difficulties should still be given verbal prompts. For although he may not be able to hear all of what is said, there is an opportunity to learn from lip movements made by the nurse.

Verbal prompts can be used in simple and complex ways. Simple verbal prompts can be used to shape up attention or carry out basic instructions like the examples above. In practice, however, where children can do what is asked of them, but cannot carry out complex behaviours on their own, a combination of verbal prompting and fading out techniques can be used to help them to learn complex tasks like choosing their own clothes and what to wear from their own wardrobe or locker. Similarly, adolescents can learn to separate out different colours, sizes, and shapes at their place of work. What these behaviours have in common is that they are all essentially sorting behaviours. Clothes are different shapes, colours, and sizes, just as many of the tasks presented to adolescents in the first early work experience presented at school, hostel, and home. If we take an example of how verbal prompting and fading-out can be used to help in learning sorting behaviour, it may be seen how the idea can be employed in a typical work task:

Example: task sorting.

Sorting task using verbal prompts and fading

Name: Carol C.

Target behaviour: to sort red, blue, and black coloured key fobs into separate piles.

Behavioural requirements for the task. Before the task is undertaken, it should be established that Carol responds to her own name and can identify red, blue, and black as different colours. She should be able to do this on verbal request. If this is not established, therapy should first be aimed at shaping up these behaviours.

Method

1. Use verbal prompts to establish sorting behaviour sequence — red, blue, black.
2. Use fading out procedure to eliminate verbal prompts, leaving sorting behaviour maintained.

This procedure is deceptively simple. It is a talk-through approach used by psychologists to help normal and handicapped children learn specific behaviours. The task is first identified. Next, it is established that the child can identify colours (notice it is not important to confuse or complicate the instruction by calling them key fobs). The child should also be able to push the coloured key fobs to the nurse on request. If any of this behaviour is absent, it should be learnt before proceeding with the next part of the task. The child should then provide desired responses to the nurse's

TABLE 8.3

Sorting task procedure:			
Therapist—verbal prompt	*Desired response for task*	*Response to prompt*	
		Correct	*Incorrect*
1. Carol, look at the colours.	Carol to look at the coloured key fobs.		
2. Push the red colours to me (it may be necessary to use a physical prompt to encourage pushing).	Carol to push red key fobs towards the nurse.		
3. Carol, give me the blue ones.	Carol to give blue key fobs to the nurse.		
4. Now give me the black ones.	Carol to give black key fobs to the nurse.		

verbal prompts. In this instance, it involves correct responses to verbal prompts 1 to 4. It is also important to record in the correct/ incorrect column if the desired behaviour occurs and when. A mark in either the correct or the incorrect column reveals how the child is responding to the task, e.g. where his performance is error free, if he gets 'stuck' on blue each time, identifies each colour properly, or does not give colours to the nurse and so on. This information can then be used to adjust the therapy programme, introduce more physical prompts with verbal prompts or break down the task into simpler steps. Whatever the alternatives are that present themselves during therapy of this kind, it should, wherever possible, be shared with nursing colleagues, the child's parents, and the other professions involved in therapy. Once all of the desired responses have been correctly and accurately learnt in the sorting behaviour, the child has then to learn to carry them out in sequence and complete the task without the aid of the nurse. The next aim for the nurse in this case, is to adopt a fading-out procedure which encourages the child to link the sequence of sorting behaviour together. The child should then perform the sorting behaviour independently of the nurse (only occasional reward should be given during the task to maintain the child's sorting behaviour, e.g. 'that's good', 'a fine job', etc.). In fading-out prompts by the nurse the following steps should be carried out:

Fading out therapist prompts (from sorting task)

1. Present all verbal prompts 1 to 4 in Table 8.3.
2. Give only verbal prompts 1 to 3.
3. Give verbal prompts 1 and 2.
4. Give verbal prompt 1.
5. Discontinue verbal prompts and occasionally reward Carol for completing sequence of sorting task behaviour.

This is a typical technique which can be used in shaping up other behaviour, such as selecting one's own clothes. It is achieved in therapy by using different combinations of physical gestural and verbal prompts.

In some instances it will be clear that the children do not maintain all of the behaviour which they have learnt during therapy. Whether this involves sorting tasks, selecting clothes, or some other learnt behaviour, such as washing their own dishes, the problem should be discussed with the therapeutic team. This should be aimed at identifying and defining where the child has difficulty in learning. For instance, the size of the fading-out steps may have been too large and therefore have to be broken down into smaller steps. Alternatively, the size of the fading-out steps may be adequate, but choice of prompts may be inappropriate, e.g. using gestural prompts alone with a visually handicapped child or failing to use both gestural and verbal prompts with the child who has impaired hearing and is learning domestic self-care and personal hygiene skills.

In practice, the nurse should aim to reduce errors of performance in the behaviour which is being learnt. By recording incorrect and correct response to therapy and dating records, useful information about the child's *learning rate* can be measured. The simplest measure of rate of learning is the *time* it takes for a child to learn new behaviour. Another measure is *how much* of any particular behaviour is learnt in each therapy session. These measures should be built into the therapy recording sheets and recorded as a matter of routine practice. Recording what goes on in therapy is one of the most vital, yet the most underestimated and overlooked areas of therapeutic management apart from the points concerning recording made in the earlier chapters, recording rates of learning is important for three reasons:

1. The therapeutic team can assess how quickly a mentally handicapped child is learning any particular target behaviour.
2. The therapeutic team can assess the appropriateness of the therapy plan being employed by the nurse (e.g. steps too large, too few prompts, sufficient number of therapy sessions, etc.).
3. The therapeutic team can consider how the rate of learning might influence the targets set for new behaviours (e.g. washing, bathing, dressing, feeding, self-catering) and the way in which new therapy plans might be formulated and put into practice.

COMMUNICATION

Another example of prompting techniques can be seen when a communication baseline is established with the mentally handicapped child. Suppose we wanted to prompt the learning of certain words in their correct context. We would do this by using different prompts and rewarding correct responses. Typical behaviours which might be learnt are connected with the words spoon, fork, knife, plate, and cup. Learning these words is important for at least two reasons: (1) the child should relate words about utensils to dining behaviour; and (2) appropriate learning of words increases the child's range of communication. A record form, like the one illustrated below, may be used to record the responses to prompts and provide a baseline assessment before beginning therapy.

Example: word learning at the dining table

Suppose we wanted to train a child to use and understand certain words in their correct *context*. You would get a base-line assessment by using different prompts and rewarding the child's correct responses. A form like the one in Fig. 8.2 is typical of what we might use to find this out. It is a useful aid for training the child.

Context: sitting at dining table

Word	'Show me your'			'Say'	'What is this'
	1	2	3	4	5
(a) Spoon					
(b) Fork					
(c) Knife					
(d) Plate					
(e) Cup					

Fig. 8.2.

(a) You would begin by holding the spoon and saying 'Johnny, what is this?'. If the child responds and says, 'Spoon', you would reinforce him and tick column 5. If the child responds incorrectly or you get no response . . .

(b) You would say, 'Johnny, say spoon'. If the child gives you the correct response tick column 4. If incorrect or no response . . .

(c) You put the spoon down amongst the other utensils and say, 'Johnny, show me the spoon'. You give no further help. If the child responds correctly tick column 3. If no response or incorrect response . . .

(d) You repeat the instruction in (c) but, at the same time, give Johnny a gestural prompt and point to the spoon. If he gets it right tick column 2. If no response or incorrect response . . .

(e) You once again repeat (c) but, at the same time, give a physical prompt to Johnny. You take his hand in yours and help him to touch the spoon.

You do this for all the words for the context in which Johnny finds himself. In this case, the dining table. An initial assessment like this lets us know which words require extra training and which only need to be repeated in the child's daily experience. The assessment also gives up the point where to begin a 'context word training programme' with the child.

Integrating skills

Integrating simply means putting together different kinds of skills that the child has learnt. For example, if a child has learnt to eat, feed himself, and sit at the table. Let us say he has also learnt how to answer to his name and carry out simple commands like: 'John, sit down', 'John, eat your dinner'. These are *two* different kinds of behaviour. One is eating/feeding behaviour, the other is responding to verbal commands or requests.

What we do in integrating skills is to get the child to learn to independently carry out combinations of behaviour wherever this is possible. So the child, as a result of useful therapeutic management, should integrate eating/feeding behaviour with verbal commands. This should also be carried out in the 'right' place at the 'right' time, e.g. the right place we would say was *in* the dining room, from food *off* a plate *on* the table. The right time is *when* the food is ready to be served (there may be exceptions to this rule, but we would only make it as a result of building it into a therapy plan.

Furthermore, not only should children integrate new skills at the right time and in the right place, they should also be shown how to mix them in the 'correct' *order*. In our example, this would mean John did not go for his dinner before the verbal request, 'John, get your dinner'. He should wait until verbally prompted, then collect his food. There are a number of other areas where we will encourage integration of different skills. These are now briefly mentioned.

FURTHER AREAS FOR INTEGRATING SKILLS

In the day-to-day use of therapy plans with children a number of integrating skills will be required of them in order for them to achieve more advanced behaviours. We have already mentioned one instance where this would apply, namely feeding and verbal commands. Here are some other areas where we would see the child beginning to integrate skills:

(1) dressing and toiletting;
(2) toy play and motor movement;
(3) toy play and communication;
(4) toy play and imitation of adults;
(5) toy play and play with adults;
(6) toy play and play with other children.

By bringing these areas of integrating skills together and getting the child to be more successful in his attempts to carry them out, we achieve more than mere integration of these simple behaviours. The child can also benefit through this approach in at least five ways.

Benefits to the child
1. The child increases the *range* of his *behaviour*.
2. The child increases the range of his experience.
3. The child has the chance to integrate together behaviour which is more complex.
4. The nurse will have helped the child to achieve more independence and *social competence*.
5. The child will have advanced in his personal development.

When we have come to the stage where we want to integrate more and more behaviours with a child, we have reached a very advanced point. Two things in the main will have happened to get to this point. These are:

1. We will have helped the child to change much of his behaviour: getting rid of undesirable behaviour and achieving desirable behaviour in various ways.
2. We will have managed to help the child to get these new behaviours or habits by observation, assessment, and planning of therapy programmes which caregivers will have carried out.

Modelling

In its simplest form, modelling means showing mentally handicapped children what it is you want them to learn. In other words, the behaviour to be learnt is demonstrated to the child. In turn, the child should then imitate the behaviour the nurse has just modelled. This is often followed with a reward which reinforces the behaviour which the child has imitated. The most common term given to learning from the modelling technique is called 'observational learning'. The child has to observe the model of behaviour the nurse presents and from it learns the behaviour expected of him.

Modelling is carried out to achieve different goals. In the first instance, behaviour can be modelled to help children learn things they could not do before. Washing, bathing, brushing teeth, and general toilet skills are typical examples. Another way of using modelling is to increase the rate of behaviour which a child has in their behaviour repertoire, but which does not happen enough or at appropriate times, e.g. helping at meal-times, learning appropriate social greetings like 'hello', 'goodbye', etc. Modelling may also be used to convey that certain behaviours results in penalties being given which have a punishing effect, e.g. dangers of handling hot liquids, food, poisonous foods, etc. Similarly, modelling a wide range of behaviours can convey rewarding consequences which result in reinforcement of the modelled behaviour, e.g. eating, switching on the television or radio, saying 'please' and 'thank you', and so on.

When modelling is used as a therapeutic technique, the nurse should not usually model the complete behaviour to be learnt. The reason for this is in the rate and quantity of behaviour that is learnt by most mentally handicapped children. They are slower than their normal contemporaries to learn behaviours like the self-help, independence, and social skills of early childhood. They never learn as quickly, nor as much in the same period of time as the normal child or adolescent, but the important point to remember is that many behaviours are learnt through modelling.

Ways of modelling

The nurse must keep the child's reduced discrimination ability in mind when planning to use modelling as a therapy technique. It must be made as clear as possible to the child what it is they are to learn, and what learning they are rewarded for. To do this, the nurse should adopt a baseline strategy to determine how modelling of any particular behaviour is to proceed. A typical assessment strategy should be concerned with providing specific answers to the following questions:

Questions to answer before proceeding with modelling

1. Has this child learnt through modelling in the past? Was it successful? Yes/No.
3. What methods were used? (specify).
4. Did this child learn as a consequence of deliberate attempt to model a specific behaviour? Was the behaviour modelled the behaviour which was learnt? If not, what behaviour was learnt instead?
5. Is there any evidence which suggests this child learns from behaviour modelled by familiar adults? (If yes, specify which ones.)
6. Is there any evidence which suggest this child learns behaviour modelled by unfamiliar adults? (If so, specify which ones.)
7. Is there any evidence which suggests this child learns behaviour modelled by familiar children? (If so, specify which ones.)
8. Is there any evidence which suggest this child learns behaviour modelled by unfamiliar children? (If so, specify which ones.)
9. Is there any evidence which suggests this child learns behaviour in familiar surroundings? (If so, specify where.)
10. Is there any evidence which suggests this child learns behaviour in unfamiliar surroundings? If so, specify where.)

This checklist procedure should reveal where some of the success and failures have occurred when and if modelling has taken place in the past. Where there is little evidence of any direct systematic attempt at modelling behaviour to the child, it should still be possible to use information from the checklist after setting up an observation assessment period. Although it may be difficult to discover what behaviours have been learnt through modelling in the absence of specific observable attempts, it can generally be assumed that a great deal of behaviour is learned in this way. The child with Down's syndrome, for instance, learns a great deal by highly accurate imitation of behaviour perceived in his surrounding. The information from the checklist procedure and discussion with a therapeutic team, should aim to define how any new behaviour is to be learnt. This means making it clear how the nurse is to model the behaviour that has to be learnt. Let us take cleaning teeth as an example and see how this might work.

Therapy model and structure of surroundings

The nurse stands next to child in tooth-brushing area. There should be a convenient waist-level sink and face-level mirror:

1. Nurse and child face mirror.
2. Child picks up toothpaste and removes cap.
3. Child picks up toothbrush (in left or right hand).
4. Holds brush against tube.
5. Squeezes tube — toothpaste on to brush.
6. Puts down tube of toothpaste.
7. Places brush against teeth.
8. Brushes (up and down or circular action).
9. Removes toothbrush from mouth.
10. Spits excess toothpaste foam out.
11. Puts toothbrush under tap and shakes it.
12. Puts toothbrush down.
13. Replaces cap on toothpaste.
14. Takes drink of water.
15. Leaves toothbrushing area.

Some practical considerations

The nurse should note the complex sequence of behaviour which has to be modelled to the child. Practical considerations should also be given to the kind of toothpaste used. The reward value of the texture, colour, and taste all affect the willingness of the child to imitate the behaviour. This is not dissimilar to the normal child who may not perform certain hygiene behaviours because he 'does not like it'. In other words, the nurse should establish if the tooth-paste itself is rewarding to the child. If it is, it is likely the tooth-brushing behaviour can be reinforced.

The next question the nurse should consider is, 'How much of the modelled behaviour is it reasonable to expect the child to learn and imitate?'. This varies from individual to individual. If the information is not available from the checklist procedure, several alternative strategies are available to test how much behaviour to model and in what way.

First, the nurse can address the child by name and say, 'Do what I do'. This should show the nurse if the child imitates the whole brushing teeth behaviour sequence after the nurse has modelled it. It was noted earlier, that modelling the complete behaviour often increases the problem of learning the prescribed behaviour for the child. An alternative strategy is to model each step of the behaviour, getting the child to imitate each step individually after the nurse. Doing this also makes it possible to observe the effects different prompts have on achieving the behaviour to be modelled. It may be sufficient to say for example, 'Emma, do this'. If she does not, a physical prompt may be necessary. In brushing teeth, the nurse is already providing gestural prompts. The response to this modelling strategy should be recorded after the period of modelling the behaviour is over. Ideally, another colleague, parent, or psychologist should record the child's response to the modelled behaviours as they occur.

Adopting this approach helps to reduce inaccuracies for the nurse when recalling how therapy progressed during the modelling period. However, it is sometimes difficult to employ it in practice because of other commitments. Although these difficulties arise, it often provides an opportunity for involving parents and other personnel in the therapy.

A third possibility is to talk the child through the behaviour as it is modelled. This talk-through approach, combined with the modelling, often promotes simultaneous learning of the behaviour — in this instance, brushing teeth. The role the mirror plays in brushing teeth is a crucial one. As the child begins to link the sequences of behaviour in brushing teeth, the behaviours will, of course, be reflected in the mirror. In effect, the child becomes their own model. The reflected behaviour acts as a stimulus to the child, promoting the next link in behaviour and so on until the sequence of tooth-brushing is completed.

Where it is clear that the child imitates models of behaviour in his surroundings, the nurse can increase the range of behaviours to be learnt. At the same time, the nurse should guard against exposing the child to models which, when learnt by imitation, lead to the so-called problem behaviours, which will have to be resolved by more therapy.

ASSIGNMENT 9

Therapy techniques

Demonstrate to each other in small groups the following therapy techniques:

(a) shaping
(b) backward chaining
(c) modelling
(d) reward presentation
(e) reward removal
(f) fading out
(g) extinction
(h) time-out training

ASSIGNMENT 10

Identify the behavioural needs to be promoted in a mentally handicapped child with whom you work. Use one or more of the therapy techniques above to achieve selected therapy targets.

9

'Problem' behaviour

DEFINING THE PROBLEM

'Problem behaviour' is also often described as 'undesirable behaviour'. Both amount to behaviour exhibited by the child which is inappropriate to his age. The presence of these behaviours renders the mentally handicapped child as 'socially unacceptable'.

There are many forms of socially unacceptable behaviour — smearing faeces, eating refuse, smashing windows, tearing curtains, etc. They can all be seen as inappropriate in one way or another. Another range of behaviour which is inappropriate is self-injurious behaviour. This presents a serious hazard to the child. Self-injuries, such as eye-gouging, self-biting, head-banging, and self-induced vomiting, can all give rise to external or internal injuries that demand medical attention. The self-injuring child is also a source of increased stress to their parents and others who care for them. Nurses, parents, and other care personnel often suffer great anxiety because they feel unable to rescue such children from the injuries which they inflict upon themselves (Bailey and Patterson 1977; Gardner 1972). However, by defining the problem behaviours, it becomes possible to intervene and reduce self-injurious behaviour and promote socially acceptable conduct.

Recording procedures should be adopted to collate relevant information about any specified problem behaviours. The nurse should also be in a position to help observers and other colleagues describe precisely the problem behaviour which requires intervention by behaviour therapy. For instance, describing a child's problem behaviour as 'poking his left eye with his right index finger' is of infinitely more practical value from a therapeutic point of view than saying the child 'gets angry with himself'. In the former case, the therapeutic team can all discuss how to carry out a detailed assessment and formulate a therapy plan. In the latter example any therapeutic team can only guess what to do next. In therapeutic management with mentally handicapped children one guess is as bad and misleading as another. Defining problems in terms of behaviours takes the guessing out of assessment and therapeutic practice. It also makes it possible to accurately record the 'problems' of the child.

EXCESSES AND DEFICITS

The problems expressed by mentally handicapped children can helpfully be seen as relative excesses and deficits of behaviour. It is important to record the excesses and deficits of behaviour should be recorded when and where they occur. Deficits of behaviour should be recorded as 'absent' when and where they are supposed to occur. Simple plus and minus charting is helpful in practice. It symbolizes plus for behaviours which are present and minus for those which are absent at the time of recording.

Repetitive handshaking and social greetings of 'hello' can be as much of a problem behaviour as having the deficit of handshaking and the accompanying hello. The same behaviour can be a problem if there is too much of it or too little. Taking excessive handshaking as an example, therapy would be aimed at reducing the handshaking, or modelling brief handshakes for the child. Alternatively, therapy may have been aimed at transforming the handshaking into waving a greeting. In this latter case, waving behaviour could also be introduced at the end of social contact — the usual 'goodbye' sign. Changing excesses of behaviour should aim to reduce, replace, or transform the behaviour that is a problem into more constructive behaviours. The one example given reveals a number of different ways in which this can be done and in different contexts using the therapy techniques discussed in the previous chapters.

Reducing excessive behaviour can be achieved by using extinction and fading-out techniques. Modified extinction and fading-out is best used where there is an *appropriate* behaviour, but too much of one, e.g. handshaking, saying 'hello', 'good morning', sitting on lap, etc. Where problem behaviours such as excessive handshaking or social greetings are highly resistant to extinction techniques, modelling competing behaviours helps to transform the problem behaviour by *maintaining* its desirable aspects. There is a vast range of problem behaviours which are excessive and inappropriate. These usually entail behaviours which are damaging to the environment and people in the environment — breaking windows or chairs, punching, biting, scratching, and the like. The self-injurious behaviours also fall into the excessive and inappropriate classification. Extinction, time-out, reward presentation (for reduction of excessive behaviour) and penalty removal for appropriate behaviour can be used effectively with this group of problems.

There is also the group of behaviours which are deficits. These may also be appropriate or inappropriate. Appropriate deficits are seen as the absence of socially unacceptable behaviour and self-injury. Where there are appropriate deficits, no therapeutic intervention is necessary. In the case of inappropriate deficits such as lack of toiletting skills, feeding, dressing, or communication and social behaviour, chaining, shaping, modelling, and prompting techniques should be introduced to help the child acquire appropriate behaviours in these areas. Modelling new behaviours in these areas of development will also be helpful for those children who can learn more quickly and greater amounts of behaviour at any time.

Many of the inappropriate deficits in the child's repertoire of behaviours will be 'wiped out' as they learn the specified target behaviours set for therapy. Each individual will learn at their own rate. In accordance with this, the nurse should pace the techniques used with the individual child. Therapy and the techniques employed to solve problem behaviours should therefore progress at the rate at which the child shows progress. Whether dealing with excesses or deficit or behaviour, the therapeutic team should be aware of the kind of problem behaviour they are attempting to resolve and the techniques to be employed in each individual case. The general guidelines in this section are set out in Table 9.1.

TABLE 9.1

Behaviours	Therapeutic techniques used
1. Excesses/appropriate	Extinction; fade-out; modelling.
2. Excesses/inappropriate	Extinction: time-out; reward presentation; penalty removal; modelling.
3. Deficits/appropriate	No therapeutic intervention required.
4. Deficits/inappropriate	Shaping prompting; chaining; and modelling.

INVESTIGATION AND IDENTIFICATION

Before the therapist can confidently arrive at a therapeutic technique or combination of techniques to put into practice with the individual child, they should have conducted a thorough investigation to identify the precise problem. The investigation of excesses and deficits of behaviour, which constitute a problem, should aim to identify three types of information. First, there should be a general estimate of excesses and deficits of behaviour. Secondly, a specific detailed assessment of any problem behaviour should be carried out. This can be done during the baseline period. Thirdly, the behaviours which have to be increased, reduced, or introduced should be made clear to parents and other caregivers.

These three types of information can be identified using Analysis of Behaviour Episode forms (ABE). These forms also provide valuable information about (1) the antecedents — what immediately preceded a behaviour; (2) the behaviour itself, the form it took; and (3) the consequences, the things which happened immediately following a behaviour episode. The antecedent, behaviour, and consequent approach to identifying problem behaviours is often referred to as the 'ABC' of identifying problem behaviour. It is not restricted to the investigation of problem behaviours however. It may be used with equal benefit to investigate and identify the occurrence of social behaviours such as polite table manners. The standard form is illustrated in Fig. 9.1.

The use of the ABE form, combined with plotting episodes on a graph during the baseline period, should be standard practice. Nurses working with parents, teachers, and social workers must ensure that no change of approach is made to the child during the baseline period. Doing this distorts the assessment of the problem behaviour and confuses the effects of intervention. There may also be extremely distressing self-injurious behaviours which can only be assessed for a short baseline period.

Example: the problem

Jenny, a girl with Down's syndrome, was 16, had partial hearing, and was completely blind. Caregives were asked to investigate the problem of self-head-punching and devise a therapy plan to reduce the problem. The ABE forms were used to identify:

(1) what started the head-punching;
(2) where Jenny was when head-punching began and ended;

Fig. 9.1.

Analysis of behaviour episode

Name: ....

Date and observer's initials	Episode began	Episode stopped	Where did it start?	Where did it stop?	What happened just before it started?	What happened just after it started?	What stopped the episode?

(3) what time episodes occurred and when they stopped;
(4) what happened during the episode; and
(5) what stopped the episode.

At the end of the baseline period, which could only be employed for 7 days, it was clear that Jenny had head-punched for two main reasons. As a result of a sudden change of environment, e.g. being moving from bedroom to lounge, lounge to playground, etc. and also to get affection from her 'mother'. In other words, Jenny had learnt to injure herself in order to gain security and contact from those who cared for her. When we consider her physical handicap in hearing and vision, combined with her severe mental handicap, this seemed one of the few effective ways to communicate her needs. However, now that Jenny's needs were recognized, the major task was to continue to fulfil them, but, at the same time, extinguish the head-punching episodes. Affection and comfort and security would also continue to be communicated to Jenny, but in a different way. A therapy was designed to achieve these goals.

The therapy plan

The therapy plan was formulated in discussion with the nurses, parents, and teachers. It had six parts — all taking the form of instructions to the nurses. It is worth listing them in full. It aimed to extinguish head-punching and reward Jenny for behaviours other than head-punching, that is socially acceptable behaviour:

1. When Jenny head-punches, wait for 5 seconds before intervening. Thereafter, extend this period to 10, 20, 30, 60 seconds, and so on. Where you have to stop the head-punching personally, try not to use your hands, but occupy Jenny's hands with a soft toy. If there is no alternative, hold Jenny's hands briskly and firmly by her sides.
2. Take toys or comforters away from Jenny when she starts head-punching. Give them to her whenever she is not head-punching. This can be done after increasing amounts of time when free from head-punching, e.g. 1, 2, 3, 4, 5 minutes, etc.
3. Give Jenny 'rough and tumble' play in periods free from head-punching. At least a morning and evening session whenever possible.
4. Fun-tickling, stroking, to be given only when head-banging is not occurring. This may be given 10-15 minutes prior to other play time.

5. Play with Jenny in lounge, kitchen, and bedroom as well as playground.
6. Toy suggestions and play: cloth animals of different textures, blocks, stroking, tickling, cuddling, rough-and-tumble wrestling.

The practice of this therapy plan by nurses, teacher, and volunteers dramatically reduced Jenny's self-injurious behaviour. It is a general approach which can be used with many other forms of self-injurious behaviour. Each therapeutic team should draw up the form that the therapy plan takes and how it is to be practised. The example shows that a combination of extinction and fading-out was used to reduce the head-punching. Reward presentation was used to increase play and socially acceptable behaviours. It also got Jenny's parents, and other people looking after her constructively involved in removing the self-injurious behaviour. As I said before, recording the episodes on a graph during the baseline period and the therapy practice is essential to get an accurate idea if the child still has the same degree of problem behaviour. A typical approach to graphing the problem behaviour episodes was used with Jenny. It is shown in Fig. 9.2.

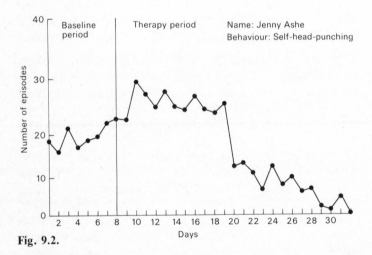

Fig. 9.2.

Jenny's graph clearly shows how she responded to therapy. As in many of the problem behaviours, there was an increase in the problem initially before the behaviour began to reduce substantially.

This is often referred to as the 'resistance effect'. It is not uncommon in normal children, adolescents, or adults. When the thing we did that worked before no longer works (gets love and affection, security, etc.), we tend to increase our attempts at the old behaviour to get the result which used to be there, but is no longer forthcoming. When an alternative behaviour can also get the same results (consequences), the old behaviour is gradually or rapidly abandoned in favour of the new alternative. One example is reducing or abandoning self-injury for love and affection in favour of play. The consequences of love and affection for the child or adolescent are still given, but for different behaviours. In Jenny's case, it was for reducing head-punching and increasing play behaviours.

Why use graphs?

In the first instance, graphs are easy to use. They provide an objective and clear picture of the problem behaviour for parents, nurses, social workers, and teachers to work on during the baseline and therapy practice phases of any therapy plan. They also provide a permanent and accurate record of problem behaviours.

Why bother when we know what the problem is?

By using graphs the problem behaviour becomes available to *anyone* involved in trying to reduce it. Without an objective and pictorial representation of the problem, everyone may 'know' what their *subjective version* of the problem is. Various versions of what a child's problem might be can be helpful and productive, but in the final analysis, it is an unbiased view of the problem behaviour which can best help. Our memories might not stretch back to a baseline period, say 30 days before therapy was practised. So graphs permit an accurate recorded memory of the problem before therapy and during its practice. Graphing also helps us to 'know', in the *objective* sense, how effectively or not we have helped a child with problem behaviours.

Do we have to take a great deal of time recording and graphing behaviour?

Graphing does not take up a great deal of time. Practice is all that is needed. Graphing also saves time in the long run. When it comes to looking back over a problem, there is an immediate record which the therapeutic team can evaluate the success of any intervention or the severity of any current problem behaviour. *Time* is, therefore, not taken up trying to remember. Parents, nurses, social workers, and teachers can get on with the job of analysing the problem behaviour episodes during the baseline and therapy practice periods.

What can graphs tell us that we don't already know?

It should be clear by now that graphs take the *effort* out of remembering and provide an accurate history of problem behaviours. They also give the present position of any problem behaviour at any particular time. Graphing shows *precisely* the episode occurrence and the relative frequency of problem behaviour. We can also tell how many episodes took place on any specific day. Elaborated graphing can also show times and places when problem behaviour took place. The Analysis of Behaviour Episode (ABE) forms can be seen as another form of graph. The main point of using any graph form is that it tells us the size of the problem behaviour to be tackled and how well we are succeeding in dealing with any specific problem behaviour. There are, therefore, good reasons for using different forms of graphing in therapy.

DIFFICULTIES DURING THERAPY

At first the parents, nurses, or teachers may experience some difficulties when practising therapy to reduce problem behaviours. Since many of the behaviours may be self-destructive or destructive to other people or objects, it may sometimes be difficult to practise the therapy plan. This may be for a number of reasons. The therapist may feel it is 'cruel' to ignore children when they are injuring themselves. Alternatively nurses themselves may feel stress. Jenny's parents, nurses, and teachers reported feeling anxious and uncomfortable at first when practising the extinction part of the therapy plan. However, it is worth reiterating that no programme should be biased towards punishment. Rewards (as in Jenny's case) should always be incorporated wherever possible to reinforce appropriate behaviour. More important though, the techniques used to reduce problem behaviours like self-injury are justified on the grounds that the child will no longer demonstrate same intensity of problem at the conclusion of therapy.

Parents may also have the greatest difficulty in employing therapy techniques which include some aspect of ignoring problem behaviour, especially the range of self-injurious behaviours. Any difficulties of the kind which can broadly be described as distressing to parents and others should be discussed with members of the therapeutic team. Finally, before proceeding with any form of therapy which involves employing and removing penalties, permission should be obtained from the child's parents or guardians. When it is not possible directly to involve parents in therapy, they should be kept up to date on the techniques being used to reduce problem behaviours and their child's response to therapy. In dealing with any form of problem behaviour which is being considered for therapeutic intervention, ethical guidelines concerning behaviour therapy techniques and their practice should always be closely followed (for example the Ethical Guidelines for the Practice of Therapy laid down by the British Association for Behavioural Psychotherapy; see also Institute of Mental Subnormality 1977).

ASSIGNMENT 11

Problem behaviour

1. Define what you mean by problem behaviour.
2. Address yourself as a team to the problem behaviour of a mentally handicapped child you are trying to help learn alternative behaviour by means of behaviour therapy.
3. Decide who should be appointed as the behaviour therapist(s).
4. Adopt appropriate therapy techniques and schedules of reinforcement and put them into practice.
5. Graph baseline period and therapy practice periods.
6. Outline your observation technique and therapeutic practice. Discuss the complete assignment with your colleagues and team supervisor/tutor.

Continuous assessment

CHECKING AND CHARTING

The previous chapters have shown how useful and important it is to assess, select targets, plan therapy, and practise therapy techniques with the mentally handicapped. This chapter emphasizes the need to have a constant check on all phases of this model. Constant checks mean evaluating the effects of each stage of therapeutic management. The therapeutic nursing process is completed by introducing a system of monitoring techniques to answer such questions as : (1) what can this child do? (2) what specific things can we teach him? (3) how shall these things be taught? (4) when will we know when they are achieved? (5) what behaviour problems are being tackled? and (6) what effect is therapy having upon any specified behaviour problems? First we can look at the ways in which assessment can be continuously evaluated.

DEVELOPMENTAL ASSESSMENT CHARTS

The developmental checklist charts (see Chapter 3), provide the basis for continuous checks on the level of development for each child. There are two main approaches in checking different aspects of development — number assessments and colour-coded assessment. The number of assessments are simply credited in the checklist each time an assessment is carried out, indicating the number of assessments for any particular person. First assessment, second assessment, third assessment, and so on. Each assessment is also dated. Colour-coded assessments are made using primary colours like red, green, and blue. A different colour is used for each assessment. For instance, red — first assessment; blue — second assessment; green — third assessment, etc. Colour notation depends upon choice, but a common code should be discussed with parents, teachers, and nursing colleagues before it is put into practice. Colour-coding should be dated at each assessment, too. An example of how number coding using 'plus' and 'minus' to indicate the pattern of development is illustrated simply in Table 10.1.

This developmental assessment checking technique helps to convey the following information on any one or combination of assessments:

(1) the general level of play development for any one assessment;
(2) the comparison between different assessments, e.g. between first, second, and third;
(3) the rate of progress in development between assessments in specific play behaviours, e.g. not playing, selecting own toys, copying play, playing with other children, etc.;
(4) suggestions for developmental teaching targets to employ in the therapy plan.

Using the developmental assessment as a checking technique allows the nurse to share with parents, teachers, and colleagues the individual way any particular child is developing. It provides an overall picture of levels of achievement between each assessment. It also makes it possible to evaluate the rate of specific areas of development for each child who has been assessed. This method of checking can be used to assess the progress of the child, both when they are receiving therapy and when they are not. It also permits the selection of different therapy targets for the child to learn as they progress in their development. For example, in the number-coded assessment above, playing alongside other children with adults', involvement/direction would be selected as the next therapy target for the child to learn. This is selected because the child has achieved most of the previous targets. Another reason for selecting this target is that it is the next most difficult behaviour to be learnt in normal development.

However, we should remember at all times that developmental charts are only helpful guides and there may be occasions when the nurse would select targets that are not always on the developmental guides. Different targets may be selected because of the child's physical handicaps. For example, learning to walk may not be considered an appropriate therapy target for a severely cerebral palsied (spastic) child. Carrying out simple verbal commands should not be

TABLE 10.1

Social play assessment

		Date: 1/7	8/9	4/12
Name: Eric Broadstair				
Play level		1	2	3

Scoring:
+ = behaviour credited
− = behaviour not credited

	Play level	1	2	3
26.	Invents own games and play for others.	−	−	−
25.	Plays games according to rules (e.g. passball, snap, rubber darts).	−	−	−
24.	Spontaneously plays with other children.	−	−	−
23.	Spontaneously plays with adults.	−	−	−
22.	Copies other children in play.	−	−	−
21.	Offers/shares toys with other children.	−	−	−
20.	Plays alongside other children without adult involvement/direction.	−	−	−
19.	Plays alongside other children with adult involvement/direction.	−	−	−
18.	Offers/shares toys with other children when adult involved.	−	+	+
17.	Requests toys or games.	−	−	+
16.	Gives toys on request.	−	+	+
15.	Offers/shares toys with adult.	−	+	+
14.	Copies adult play without need for prompting.	—	—	+
13.	Copies adult play after prompting (using physical, gestural, or verbal prompts).	−	+	+
12.	Keeps toys to himself.	+	+	+
11.	Can find duplicate toy from bag of toys.	−	+	+
10.	Can discover toy you hide behind your back or screen.	+	+	+
9.	When toy is taken away child will physically search for it.	+	+	+
8.	When toy is taken away child looks for it with eyes.	+	+	+
7.	When toy is taken away child shows no further interest.	+	+	+
6.	Throws toys away and doesn't look for them.	+	+	+
5.	Uses toy to hit other objects or people.	+	+	+
4.	Puts toys to mouth (sucks, bites, etc.).	+	+	+
3.	Selects own toys.	+	+	+
2.	Toys selected for child.	+	+	+
1.	Shows interest in toys but does not play.	+	+	+
0.	Does not play (e.g. sits or lies around).			

Relevant observations: Eric has shown a gradual increase in the range of his play behaviours between assessment intervals. Discuss the possibility of planning therapy for Eric to learn target no. 19 — playing alongside other children with adult involvement/direction.

expected of deaf children. However, in the latter example, it may be possible if accompanies with sign language or easily understood gestures (Walker 1980).

MONITORING THERAPY PRACTICE

Once a therapy plan has been selected, it should be monitored closely when it is put into practice. The nurse should be concerned with helping the mentally handicapped to fulfil their needs and promote their development. The best way to achieve this aim is, firstly to know what it is that has to be monitored, and secondly, to have a method for recording what the therapeutic team have decided to monitor. In the first instance, this may be a concrete target such as finding out if a child can learn to plant potatoes in his parents' garden, cut the grass, and perform other garden skills. This might also be part of a wider programme entailing life survival skills such as cooking and personal hygiene. Whatever the targets, the nurse should concern themselves with monitoring at least five aspects of therapy. This can be constituted as a 'monitoring panel'.

The monitoring panel

Before practising any therapy, a monitoring panel like the one shown below, can be drawn up. This allows the nurse to report back to parent and colleagues on the child's progress.

Five-point panel

(1) Monitor the number of therapy sessions carried out (this may be done by counting and may include the length of time spent by the nurse on each session);
(2) Monitor the number of therapy sessions taken to achieve therapy targets with each child;
(3) What therapeutic techniques were used to achieve therapy targets?
(4) What rewards and/or penalties were employed during therapy?
(5) Which therapists are involved in employing the therapy plan?

This approach is an essential part of therapy. Its main advantage is that it gives the nurse an effective and responsible co-ordinating opportunity to involve parents, teachers, social workers, and other colleagues at the most important point of therapy — its practice. Co-ordinating information from the therapy plan, as it is practised, also permits the nurse to occupy a controlling function in therapy.

This function is concerned with regularly assessing and reviewing the efficacy and appropriateness of any therapy for each child. The co-ordinating and control functions of monitoring therapy and its practice are best done by working as 'teams of therapists', rather than as isolated caregivers. In general, it helps for 'everyone' to know what is going on in therapy and what results are appearing from its practice. This is helpful because a common framework for discussion therapy and its practice is established. It does not mean that members of any therapeutic team connected with therapy practice need always agree with the way in which a therapy plan has been chosen or is being employed, but it rightly takes the ambiguity out of therapeutic discussion. It will however eventually facilitate agreement about therapeutic goals — how they are to be practised and who is to practise them. The monitor panel method is one way of promoting 'good' therapeutic practice and teamwork. Figure 10.1 shows an example of how the panel can be incorporated into a standard recording form (similar working records can be designed to monitor problem behaviour; the ABC method of recording is another example (see p.102)).

Using the Therapy Monitoring Panel it becomes possible to make a routine check of all the stages of therapy, while it is being practised. The nurse can also share the information from the monitoring record with parents and colleagues. It also provides the information on which future therapy plans can be based, and current monitoring can be related to the five-point panel.

In the example shown in Fig. 10.1, we can see that 'Caroline' has been learning the target behaviour 'washing hair'. The nurse's record shows that:

(1) she has received 27 therapy sessions to date, each of 10 minutes' duration;

(2) she has taken 23 therapy sessions to begin to show signs of learning the therapy target 'washing own hair';

(3) modelling and verbal and physical promptings were employed as therapy techniques;

(4) the rewards used were rose-perfumed soap (Caroline liked various perfumes) and looking at herself in the mirror when her hair was dried after washing. Penalties consisted of reward removal, e.g. removing the soap or the mirror if Caroline refused to complete washing;

(5) two therapists were involved: Caroline's mother and the community nurse (the community nurse showed the mother how to score the therapy session given on the monitoring record).

Fig. 10.1.

Therapy monitoring panel

Name: *Caroline Smith* Sex: *F* Chronological age: *15* Date begun: *1 August 1981*	

Diagnosis:.. Associated ....
..........*Severely Mentally*.......... problems: *Lacks basic personal*........
..........*Handicapped*.......... ....*hygiene skills*....................

Behaviour goal (s)	A *Hairwashing*	C	
	B	D	

Programme steps	(i) Modelling (ii) Verbal prompts (iii) Physical prompts
What to do	(a) Caregiver shows Caroline wash area and stands beside her (b) Model gradual step-by-step complete hairwash (c) Each step is supported by 'Caroline do this'
Where and when	Therapy sessions to be carried out in bathroom of parent's house between 8 p.m. and 8.30 p.m.
How often	Three times per week on alternate evenings. Change the evenings each week. e.g. Mon, Wed, Fri / Tues, Sat, Sun
Personal rewards to use as reinforcers	1. Rose-perfumed soap to smell and wash face with after hairwash. 2. Looking at herself in bathroom mirror after hairwash and whilst washing face	* Remember to reward with a 'reinforcer' immediately child/young adult has succeeded with the behaviour goal.

Date. Now tick the therapy session below in the correct date box.

1 ✓	2 ✓	3 ✓	4 ✓	5 ✓	6 ✓	7 ✓	8 ✓	9 ✓	10 ✓	
11 ✓	12 ✓	13 ✓	14 ✓	15 ✓	16 ✓	17 ✓	18 ✓	19 ✓	20 ✓	
21 ✓	22 ✓	23 ✓	24 ✓	25 ✓	26 ✓	27 ✓	28	29	30	31

Tick box when behaviour
goals achieved and circle
letter when behaviour
goals established

Behaviour goal			
ⓐ	b	c	d

Tick box for period of follow-up assessment	1 week	4 weeks	1 month	2 months ✓	3 months
	4 months	5 months	6 months	9 months	12 months

Therapist's names	1	*Evelyn Smith (mother)*
	2	*David Crown (community nurse)*
	3	

The therapy Monitoring Panel can be used in its present form or adapted by any therapeutic team to monitor specific areas of a child's development. As we have seen, the most effective way of employing it is to set therapy targets which can be observed and monitored in therapeutic practice. Setting behaviour which can be promoted using the various therapy techniques discussed earlier (see Chapter 7). The nurse not only knows what is going on in therapy, but also if it is effective and appropriate for each individual. In other words, nurses have control over the therapy which is being practised. This control should always be directed at fulfilling the psychological and developmental needs of each child, and since a basic need of children — whether handicapped or otherwise — is the need to achieve a sense of personal recognition, any therapeutic effort must take into account each person's likes and dislikes.

Recognizing the 'likes and dislikes' of each child amounts to understanding his idea of rewards and penalties. In endeavouring to find out the 'likes and dislikes' of each child we recognize and appreciate the child for themselves. We also have the opportunity of discovering rewards and penalties which can be incorporated into therapy plans and used to achieve therapeutic success. Monitoring personal likes and dislikes is therefore an essential procedure of effective therapeutic management. It should also be considered as a basic principle of behaviour therapy.

PERSONAL 'LIKES' AND DISLIKES'

Periodic and regular assessment of what each child likes and dislikes is a critical part of therapeutic nursing practice. Just as normal children change their tastes, so, too, do the mentally handicapped. From the point of view of therapeutic management, the nurse can usefully conceptualize likes and dislikes into rewards and penalties. It is helpful to know what acts as rewards for each individual child and what has penalizing effects. As we have seen earlier, what may act as a reward for one child, e.g. ice cream, nuts, fruit, tickling, etc., may have the effect of a penalty for another (see Chapter 5). The main reason for periodic assessment of likes and dislikes is that it effects what rewards are to be used as potential reinforcers during therapy. Nursing therapists will get 'better' therapeutic results by employing a therapy plan which incorporates rewards the child likes very much.

THE PERSONAL REWARD PROFILE

A simple and effective way of assessing likes and dislikes is to chart an individual's personal reward profile. Look at the personal reward profile (Fig. 10.2) which has been employed and shows the range of likes and dislikes of 'Sharon' a 14-year-old, severely mentally handicapped teenager.

The very strong likes were used as rewards in the therapy plan which was drawn up for her. It was a feeding plan which only began to show progress after the most attractive 'likes' had been identified on the reward profile. Periodical assessment of her likes and dislikes showed some variation. This was accounted for in slight changes by incorporating the new reward preferences into the feeding plan and dropping previous ones which were no longer therapeutically effective. Failure to identify appropriate likes and dislikes can be avoided by systematic and period assessment. Constructing and monitoring a personal reward profile is another effective way of providing accurate information about how tastes change over time. The practical value of personal reward profiling lies in selecting and monitoring the effectiveness of rewards employed during the course of therapy.

THERAPEUTIC FAILURE

Some therapy may fail to achieve the selected learning targets. This is not an event which is exclusive to cases where therapy is carried out by nurses. We only have to look at the case-notes of mentally handicapped people in residential care to see the numbers of changes in so-called therapeutic approaches. These often reflect no corresponding progress in the development of the mentally handicapped, but merely a juggling of organizational resources, or transfer to different 'therapy' departments, such as adopting medication and medication measures. On these actions there is little evidence of fulfilling the needs of the mentally handicapped persons. Equally important, there are few baseline measures taken to compare the efficacy of any therapy with the outcome they produce, e.g. if hyperactivity has been observed in a mentally handicapped child, what specific effects does a tranquillizer like Largactil, or a central nervous stimulant like Ritalin have upon the hyperactive behaviour? The same can be said of poly-medication and social education practices. It is clear that failure to help the mentally handicapped to fulfil their needs and promote their

Fig. 10.2.

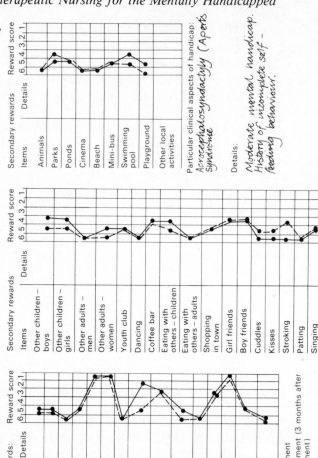

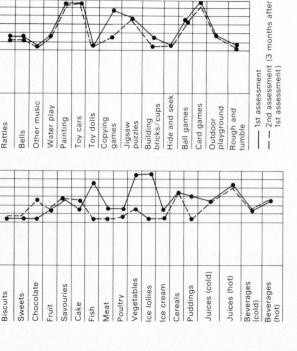

PERSONAL REWARD PROFILE

Name: *Sharon White*
Age: *14 years*

Scoring
1. Don't know 2. No opportunity 3. Very unrewarding
4. Unrewarding 5. Rewarding 6. Very rewarding

Primary rewards

Items	Details	Reward score
Biscuits		
Sweets		
Chocolate		
Fruit		
Savouries		
Cake		
Fish		
Meat		
Poultry		
Vegetables		
Ice lollies		
Ice cream		
Cereals		
Puddings		
Juices (cold)		
Juices (hot)		
Beverages (cold)		
Beverages (hot)		

Secondary rewards:

Items	Details	Reward score
Rattles		
Bells		
Other music		
Water play		
Painting		
Toy cars		
Toy dolls		
Copying games		
Jigsaw puzzles		
Building bricks/cups		
Hide and seek		
Ball games		
Card games		
Outdoor playground		
Rough and tumble		

———— 1st assessment
– – – – 2nd assessment (3 months after 1st assessment)

Secondary rewards

Items	Details	Reward score
Other children – boys		
Other children – girls		
Other adults – men		
Other adults – women		
Youth club		
Dancing		
Coffee bar		
Eating with others – children		
Eating with others – adults		
Shopping in town		
Girl friends		
Boy friends		
Cuddles		
Kisses		
Stroking		
Patting		
Singing		

Secondary rewards

Items	Details	Reward score
Animals		
Parks		
Ponds		
Cinema		
Beach		
Mini-bus		
Swimming pool		
Playground		
Other local activities		

Particular clinical aspects of handicap:
Acrocephalosyndactyly (Aperts Syndrome

Details:
Moderate mental handicap.
History of incomplete self –
feeding behaviour.

development is not restricted to the practice of therapeutic nursing. However, by adopting a systematic approach towards therapy, the nurse can monitor the different processes of assessment, therapy, and continuous assessment. The monitoring of these processes should constructively and clearly show where therapeutic progress is being made and also where therapeutic failure is specifically evident.

We shall concentrate on identifying therapeutic failure here, since therapeutic progress has been dealt with earlier.

IDENTIFYING THERAPEUTIC FAILURE

Identifying therapeutic failure should always be aimed at rectifying any aspect of therapeutic nursing which prevents the achievement of therapeutic goals. This is a principle which many other forms of therapy would also uphold. However, like other therapies, e.g. drug therapy, speech therapy, physiotherapy, and art therapy, it is often difficult, whether working individually or in a team, to detect the precise source of therapeutic failure. This is one of the weaknesses of the therapies in general under our current state of knowledge in mental handicap. Therapeutic management, therefore, like the other therapies employed in mental handicap, has to account for and identify:

(1) general failures or behaviour therapy;
(2) specific failures of behaviour therapy;
(3) the reasons why general and specific failures may have occurred in behaviour therapy (this is a prerequisite to rectifying, where possible, 'faulty' therapeutic management).

How is this achieved? By addressing ourselves to the nursing process employed in therapeutic management. Failure of therapeutic nursing should be reflected in the way the nurse and the therapeutic team have carried out their observations, assessments, therapy target selections, therapy planning, and therapy monitoring tasks. There is no one formula for detecting specific therapeutic failures in the sense that when a therapy target is not achieved it will always be the same cause. For instance, failure to learn to feed, dress, groom, and exchange social graces — 'good morning', 'good-bye' — may have the same causes or different causes. The formula that can be applied is that which the therapeutic management approach to behaviour therapy permits — namely that of checking and reassessing each part of the process the nurse has previously carried out.

Keeping scrupulous and meticulous records of each stage of therapeutic management employed by nurses is essential if we are to begin to identify the specific causes of therapeutic failure.

Although there is often no obvious straight cause-effect relationship between therapeutic failure and its cause(s), there are some important guidelines and checks to make when it occurs. These are briefly outlined in the Therapeutic Failure Detection Guide (Table 10.2).

THERAPEUTIC FAILURE DETECTION GUIDE

This guide can be used when failure to achieve therapeutic goals is evident. Usually, it is important to start off by stating the general nature of the failure and then consider specific aspects of the therapeutic strategy which might elucidate the exact source of the failure for any particular child. The failure does not rest with the child, but with the nurse and therapeutic team who are responsible for designing and carrying out successful therapeutic management. The guide is one which not only helps the individual therapist to evaluate therapy but is also useful in discussion with parents, school, and other hospital personnel, who may be directly involved in the therapeutic team.

TABLE 10.2

Therapeutic failure detection guide

Name. Sex. Age. Description of mental and physical handicaps. General failure. characteristics. (This may be a statement as general as 'has not made progress', etc.)

Specific failure	Characteristics	Agree/Disagree (Tick appropriate one)
Observation	Initial observations made for too short a period (i.e. baseline measure inadequate)	
	Wrong method of observation employed (i.e. time-interval as opposed to episode observation)	
	Behaviour observed was inconsistent with that agreed in therapeutic team	
Assessment*	Selected inappropriate developmental scale or other method of assessment	
	Did not score the assessment of person according to the scale manual	
	Did not take account of additional handicaps (e.g. degree of cerebral palsy, spasticity)	
	Did not consider other psychological needs (see Chapter 1)	

Specific failure	Characteristics	Agree/Disagree (Tick appropriate one)
Therapy target selection	Did not make a team decision on therapy target priorities Did not consider the complexity of the therapy target(s) selected for therapy Did not consider the utility value for the child (e.g. if learning to draw a circle is of practical value for him to learn)	
Therapy formulation	Did not include other relevant people in therapy plan (e.g. parents, teachers, etc.) Omitted to include rewards the child liked very much into the therapy plan Set unrealistic review dates to assess person's response to the therapy plan (e.g. setting a bi-weekly review date to assess therapeutic 'progress' instead of bi-monthly review dates)	
Therapeutic practice	Selection of therapy techniques not discussed with therapeutic team Therapist(s) not skilled in selected therapy techniques to be practised Therapy techniques not suited to learning style of individual, e.g. selected modelling when step-by-step shaping is required Did not practise the therapeutic techniques selected and decided by therapeutic team	
Continuous assessment	Omitted to record initial observations Did not record all stages of the assessment Inadequate baseline period information Insufficient monitoring and recording of therapy session (e.g. failing to record a session which was carried out or recording as carried out, a session which was not) Did not check on possible changes in likes and dislikes on the Personal Reward Profile Review not carried out at interval set by therapeutic team (e.g. review conducted before review date)	

*The exception is where the mentally handicapped child or adolescent is physically ill.

Any one of these failures or any combination of them may be responsible for a failure of therapeutic management. When a therapeutic failure does occur, the nurses and the therapeutic team should carry out the detection guide checking procedure. The information available can then be analysed. The source or sources of therapeutic failure can then be detected and identified. The detection of specific failures in therapeutic management using this guide are by no means exhaustive, but the guide serves as a constructive clinical tool which will be sufficient to identify many of the failures which may occur in the nurse's employment of therapeutic nursing.

Finally, the Detection Guide should also be used as an aid to *rectifying* therapeutic failure. For instance, if in Therapy Formulation rewards which the child did not 'like' very much were included in the therapy plan, these should be replaced by more effective 'likeable' ones.

If we take one other example from therapeutic practice, the rectifying value of the Detection Guide is evident. Nurses who do not have the necessary skills to carry out a therapy plan should receive appropriate training in these therapy techniques. Therapeutic failure in behavioural therapy is, therefore, amenable to constructive investigation using different stages of therapeutic management. The concept of the therapeutic management also permits this practice investigation with a view to rectifying therapeutic failures. It requires a disciplined approach to behaviour therapy as well as a clear appreciation of the concept of the nurse's role in therapeutic nursing.

ASSIGNMENT 12

1 . Carry out a team developmental assessment.
2. Select therapy targets to put into therapeutic practice.
3. Draw up the therapy monitoring panel.
4. Monitor therapeutic practice.
5. Evaluate personal likes and dislikes prior to and during therapy.
6. Discuss the effectiveness of therapy and any failures against the therapeutic failure detection guide.
7. Conduct the assignment involving parents, social workers, and nurses.
8. Present the assignment for discussion under the supervision of your team tutor.

11

A model for therapeutic management

INTEGRATING THERAPEUTIC PRACTICE

The various phases of therapeutic nursing outlined in the earlier chapters can now be integrated into a practical therapeutic model. The sequences of assessment and observation, therapy formulation, therapeutic practice and continuous evaluation permit the nurse to carry out systematic therapy. Each part of this sequence is related to the other. For therapeutic management to be effective no part of the sequence or stages in the therapeutic process should be omitted. For example, it would be unhelpful to decide on the therapeutic techniques to use *before* assessing, observing, and selecting the therapy targets a child might learn. Another point to keep in mind is that although each stage of the nursing process is carried out independently, it is with a view to preparing for the next stage and so on. The model for therapeutic management illustrated in Fig. 11.1 shows how caregiver therapy is practised.

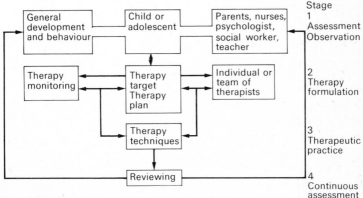

Fig. 11.1. Therapeutic management model.

The model shows how the different stages of therapeutic management reflect a number of complex psychological processes, which the caregiver can conduct as therapy progresses. This model is also one way of integrating the involvement of parents, nurses, psychologists, social workers, and teachers who may be involved in any therapeutic effort. Therapeutic management as portrayed in this model can be used to connect theory and practice when working with the mentally handicapped. The theory is necessary for a clear understanding as to which stage of the therapeutic process should be carried out in practice. Conversely, any specific aspect of therapeutic management should reflect which part of the therapeutic process is being carried out in practice.

In its simplest form, the nurse should be guided by the model as to what stage of the therapeutic process to practise in therapeutic management. Similarly, the particular aspect of practice informs the nurse what stage of therapy is being carried out at any one time during therapeutic practice. An example shows how the model of therapeutic management might be used in practice.

Example

The caregiver has been asked to carry out therapeutic nursing with Frances, an 11-year-old severely mentally handicapped girl. Frances has been described as 'a problem child', who picks her skin all the time. She attends school and lives at home with her parents.

This example is typical of the scanty and generally vague information that many nurses, parents, teachers, social workers, and psychologists have to work from. It is obvious that it is insufficient, ambiguous, and largely unhelpful. The application of therapy specifically designed to promote learning and consider the needs of the mentally handicapped child, cannot be achieved using this approach. However, by employing the therapeutic process outlined in the therapeutic management model, clear information can be identified which is of practical benefit to the nurse, parent, and others who are engaged in therapy. We can now see how this vague approach to therapy with the mentally handicapped can be transformed into clear, intelligible, and practically useful information to carry out effective caregiver therapy with cases like Frances.

Therapeutic process: stage one

Adopting the stage by stage approach outlined in the model, the following individual developmental and behavioural profile was mapped out for Frances. It was done by the community nurse, parents, and teachers.

Assessment and observation of behaviour episodes

Behaviour. The community nurse and Frances's parents agreed to observe and record the number of skin-picking episodes at home. The Analysis of Behaviour Episode forms were used. It was found that there was no need to observe skin-picking at school as it did not occur there. However, with the permission of the parents, all the findings of the ABE forms were shared with the schoolteacher. The analysis of behaviour episode forms revealed the information given in Table 11.1.

TABLE 11.1

Analysis of behaviour

Definition of problem: Skin-picking

Location:	Home	School
Frequency:	15	Nil

	Picking	Not picking
Number of times observed using 3-minute observation periods = 100 observations	15	75
Father present	0	100
Mother present	15	75
Father and mother present	0	100

Further analysis showed that at the weekends (when father was home) there was only one isolated skin-picking episode. The community nurse deduced from this evidence — collected over a period of five weeks — that the absence of father for long periods of time was a central factor in Frances's skin-picking behaviour. This was shared with the parents and the school teacher. The nurse could now use the information from stage one of the therapeutic process and proceed to stage two. This stage, as you may remember from the model of the therapeutic management, involves the formulation of therapy.

Therapeutic process: Stage two

During this stage, therapy targets are selected, therapists are identified and the way therapy is to be monitored is made clear. Put this together amounts to the therapy plan.

Therapy formulation

Therapy target: Reduce or extinguish skin-picking behaviour.

Team of therapists
(a) Mr and Mrs Fairweather.
(b) Sally Brown — schoolteacher.
(c) Dorothy Simpson — community nurse.

Monitoring of therapy This stage of the therapeutic process would enlist all or some of the monitoring points mentioned earlier in the five-point monitor panel. In Frances's case the community nurse, parents, and teachers were all interested to find out if the problem behaviour could be overcome in eight weeks. This figure was transformed into 40 days as no skin-picking episodes occurred at weekends. All of the five points in the therapy monitoring panel were adopted. Rewards of Frances's liking were also selected for the therapy plan using the personal reward profile and information from the ABE. The therapy plan is outlined in Table 11.2.

The simulated findings of the therapy plan which is typical of an actual case can be presented quite clearly on a therapy graph (Fig. 11.2).

ANALYSIS OF THERAPEUTIC NURSING
Therapeutic process: Stage three

The therapy plan and graph information should help the nurse to analyse the effects of practising therapeutic management. This can be done most clearly by relating the findings of any case to the therapeutic process outlined in the model of therapeutic management. It provides a series of cross checks which helps the therapeutic team to focus on the value of their co-operative intervention. If we take the above case as an example, the nurse, parents, and teacher were able to analyse both the baseline period and the therapeutic practice period for evidence of skin-picking.

Agreement, between them came from the evidence of the therapy plan and the graph recordings. Any opinions and judgements about Frances's skin-picking therefore flowed from her *behaviour* and not vague unobservable, notions such as 'psychotic episode' or unhelpful psychiatric diagnostic labels. Describing, and recording described beaviour is the first step in behaviour analysis.

TABLE 11.2

Therapy plan

Names: Frances Fairweather   **Chronological age:** 11 years
Date therapy began: 1/6/81
Diagnosis: Severe mental handicap
Associated problems: Self-mutilation skin-picking
Therapy target: Reduce or extinguish skin-picking
Rewards to employ: Presence of father
                      Talking of father in father's absence
                      Photograph of father
Monitoring therapy: Record each therapy session given. Enter whether or not
                      skin-picking episode occurred by 'E' otherwise leave blank.

The next stage of the therapeutic process is the normal practice of caregive therapy and involves the therapy techniques to employ with the therapy plan.

Therapy techniques: Combine reward presentation for all skin-picking-free
                      episodes with reward removal for skin-picking episodes.
                      When rewards and penalties lead to signs of appropriate
                      behaviour (i.e. reduction in skin-picking). Fade out
                      presence of father but maintain talking about father and
                      presenting photograph at variable intervals.
Recording: Record each therapy session and any problem behaviour
                      episode.
Reviewing: Review observations and assessment of skin-picking behav-
                      iour. Discuss with parents and teacher. Present number of
                      therapy sessions carried out using therapy techniques and the
                      response to therapy. Draw up a therapy graph showing base-
                      line assessment and response to caregiver therapeutic prac-
                      tice. Share findings and plan any new therapeutic strategy
                      with parents and teacher. Take into consideration any change
                      in Frances's behaviour and pattern of psychological needs.

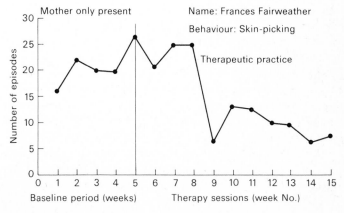

Fig. 11.2.

By adopting this disciplined approach, the nurse, teacher, and Frances's parents were able to analyse what had happened before and during therapy with Frances. Considering the case through the sequence of the process the found:

1. Frances had a problem which could be identified and best be described in behavioural terms as 'skin-picking'.
2. The baseline period assessment should be carried out for 5 weeks prior to any therapy.
3. Baseline period assessment revealed skin-picking behaviour only occurred in the absence of Frances's father.
4. The therapy target should be a reduction in skin-picking and possible elimination of the behaviour.
5. The therapy formulation for the therapy plan should involve carrying out therapy at home.
6. Response to therapy would be monitored and recorded by Frances's parents. Findings would be shared with the school-teacher.
7. The therapeutic techniques would consist of (1) reward presentation (2) reward removal, and (3) fade-out procedures.
8. Reviewing should take into consideration the response to therapeutic practice.
9. Therapeutic practice should be carried out for a period of 10 weeks.
10. Any further assessment, observation, target setting, planning-practising of therapy and reviewing should be pursued employing the therapeutic process within the model of therapeutic management.

RESPONSE TO THERAPY

Therapeutic process: Stage four

The response to therapy should ideally be analysed at the end of the period set for therapy sessions. However, in practice, the nurse will be able to get some idea of how therapy is progressing. Sometimes this is very useful in that it encourages the parents, nurse, and other colleagues to maintain their therapeutic effort. On the other hand, apparently worsening results can lead to a false sense of personal inadequacy on the part of the various therapists.

The case presented here to illustrate the model of therapeutic management and the therapeutic process in practice, shows how misleading premature decisions about the way therapy is going can be made. For instance, if the therapists working with Frances thought they would meet to analyse her response to therapy after week number 7 or 8, they would find the response to therapy had resulted in an *increase* in the skin-picking behaviour. If this was then compared with the baseline period assessment weeks 1, 2, 3, and 4, it may also seem that therapeutic practice using this particular therapy plan is not helping Frances. However, comparison with week 5 of baseline would show some improvement for the therapeutic practice period sessions throughout the *whole* of the time the therapy plan was in operation.

The point to notice here is that analysis of the response to therapy in any case of therapeutic management should take into close consideration the complete patterning of specified behaviour before, during, and at the completion of pre-defined set of therapy sessions. Otherwise, many of the conclusions reached about any therapeutic endeavour may be premature and misleading. A practical consequence of premature analysis of response to therapy may lead to undue disappointment in parents, teachers, and nurses. Premature analysis of response to therapy can, and often does, lead to premature closures of therapeutic practice. When this happens, it may serve against the interests and needs of the child. Remembering that learning should progress at the rate which the child proceeds is one guideline to maintaining or early termination of therapeutic practice. It is preferable though, to carry out the prescribed number of therapy sessions detailed in the therapy plan. When this is done, any questions regarding the suitability of the entire plan or its parts can be made. The number of therapy sessions conducted with the child could then be just one question among many to be raised in the analysis of response to therapy. Other questions may be relevant too; such as, should we consider adding to, reducing, or changing the rewards to be used in reinforcement and punishment? Another crucial question in analysing response to therapy concerns the targets set for therapy. In Frances's case 'reduce or extinguish skin-picking' was the target to aim for in therapeutic practice. The therapy target is often referred to as the 'criterion' for the therapeutic success. Criteria set for therapy plans can either be 'loose' or 'tight'.

This just means they can be highly specific or more general. In Frances's case a reduction in skin-picking did occur for the overall therapeutic practice period. This was the general behaviour profile reflected in observer recordings. However, the recordings are also more specific. They also show the number of episodes of skin-picking per week and between weekly therapy sessions. The response to therapy indicated here is more detailed. The criterion for analysing the response to therapy is in this sense tighter. It would have been possible to make it even tighter. For instance, it could have been written into the therapy plan that both baseline and therapy sessions would be 'carried out daily at 2 p.m.'.

The response to therapy as it is shown in Frances's case shows a general trend of reduction in skin-picking — one of the criteria for therapeutic success. However, the optimal target, extinguishing skin-picking, has not been achieved during the time period allocated for therapeutic nursing using the particular therapy plan designed for Frances. The nurse, parents, and teacher concluded that the therapy plan should continue for another 8 weeks since there was clear evidence of a steady decline in the problem behaviour.

THE FUTURE

Working with the model of therapeutic nursing, and the sequences of the process outlined in the earlier chapters, the nurse can equip herself to carry out effective therapy with mentally handicapped children. It should be clear that this introduction to therapeutic nursing is also an attempt to whet the appetite of nurses to take an active part in the therapeutic process. The application of therapeutic nursing in mental handicap provides a welcome change from drug-oriented therapy. The application of therapeutic nursing in mental handicap has already been used to promote development in children and adolescents to good effect. Many studies have also shown how effective the processes of assessment, observation, target therapy planning, and therapeutic practice have been in rectifying problem behaviours in the mentally handicapped. Much of this work has been done by psychologists to date. However, there is now a growing need for nurses to take up the challenge of therapeutic nursing and apply it to the problems they consider important to resolve in their work with the mentally handicapped and their families. The psychological approach to therapeutic nursing outlined here should make it possible for nurses to work in the first in stance as co-therapists with psychologists in the field of mental handicap. However, the logical outcome of therapeutic nursing is for nurses to become largely independent therapists and to work in a team. This is a great hope. It is the nurse-therapist, working in partnership with parents and others, who will transform this hope into a working reality. When this has been achieved therapeutic nursing for the mentally handicapped should have become established as an important development in the theory and practice of nursing.

ASSIGNMENT 13

1. Carry out a complete investigation with a mentally handicapped child employing all stages of the therapeutic management model. You will remember there are four main stages in the model:
   (a) observation and assessment
   (b) therapy formulation
   (c) therapeutic practice
   (d) continuous assessment.

   This assignment should be carried out by the team members under supervision. A problem behaviour may be tackled or any of the developmental areas shown on the developmental scales. A full and detailed account of the assignment should be shared with colleagues, parents, social workers, teachers, and where possible with the mentally handicapped child who has received the assessment and therapy. Discussion of the overall therapeutic strategy should be conducted by the supervisor-tutor of those personnel in training.

ASSIGNMENT 14

1. Conduct an individual assignment similar to Assignment 12.
2. Evaluate the advantages and disadvantages of individual and team assignments under the model of therapeutic management.

ASSIGNMENT 15

1. Present a full and complete account of the nursing approach to therapeutic management in mental handicap.

   (This final assignment exercise can be done in teams or individually. The assignment can draw on actual work you have carried out yourselves as nurse-therapists as well as drawing on other sources of information and practice.)

   Finally as in the previous assignments, the account — whether presented in writing or using audio-visual aids — should be discussed with your supervisor-tutor and members of your training team.

Thank you for working through this book and attempting these therapeutic management assignments. You should now be in a position, with the help of your colleagues and supervisors, to assess the contribution you may be able to make to therapeutic nursing with the mentally handicapped.

Appendix 1

Some clinical conditions associated with mental handicap

Condition	Causes	Clinical features
Acrocephalosyndactyly (Apert's syndrome)	Dominant gene	Commonest features abnormally high head, degree of fusion of digits. Associated with paternal age. Rare. Degree of mental handicap variable.
Agenesis	Congenital	Malformation during foetal growth. Brain may be underdeveloped. May be both mental and physical retardation.
Amaurotic family idiocy (cerebromacular degeneration) e.g. Tay-Sachs disease	Single recessive gene Disorder of lipid metabolism	Most affects Jewish race. Normal development until about 3 months, then overt signs general weakness, spasticity, muscle wasting, in addition to degeneration of nerve cells. Death usually within 4 years of onset. 'Cherry-red' spot on retina. Rare condition, Tay-Sachs disease is commonest form. No treatment.
Anoxia	Birth trauma	Malformation of placenta. Pre-eclamptic toxaemia. Prolonged second stage of labour. Varying degrees of subnormality.
Autism	Neurological, but specifics unknown	Often combined with subnormality and adds to retardation. 'Hypnotic' preoccupation with limited range of stimuli, communication difficulties, lack of affect, may exhibit good motor skills and feats of memory.
Bloch-Sulzberger syndrome	Probably due to mutant gene with sex limitation	Usually manifest soon after birth, but may be up to fourth year. Anomaly in pigment distribution, and may be epilepsy and microcephaly. Mainly affects females. Often associated with mental retardation, which may be severe.

Condition	Causes	Clinical features
Cerebral palsy	Birth trauma Sometimes recessive gene defect	Neurological damage, usually affecting motor movements, hemiplegia, quadriplegia, and many are epileptic. Commonly associated with varying degrees of mental handicap.
Congenital rubella syndrome	Rubella contracted within first three months of pregnancy	May cause mental handicap, deafness, cataract and heart disease. Reduction in incidence due to availability of vaccination.
Congenital syphilis	Treponema pallidum organism infects infant via placental membrane	Infant fails to thrive. Shows rash on skin and lesions around mouth, anus, genitals. Involvement of nervous system may include convulsions, hydrocephalus. Antisyphilitic treatment essential.
Craniostenosis	Premature fusion of cranial sutures	Malformation of skull with secondary effects on CNS.
Cretinism	Disorder of endocrine metabolism (thyroxin deficiency)	Appears around 6 months. Baby shows rather coarse skin, thin hair, lethargy. Usually thyroid treatment effective.
Cri-du-chat syndrome (Cat cry)	Abnormality of chromosome 5	Characteristic cat-like cry. Physical abnormalities, slanted eyes, small, head, abnormalities of ears and mouth. Severe mental handicap.
Diabetes mellitus	Ante-natal toxic infection	Skin pigmentation, lethargy, coma. Cases of subnormality, but susceptible to insulin treatment.
Down's syndrome (Mongolism)	Chromosome abnormality (Trisomy 21/22)	Physical features: small round head, slant eyes, straight hair, web fingers, thick lips. Moderate-severe retardation. Longevity reduced.
Echolalia	Congenital organic impairment	Malfunction of left hemisphere. Often associated with subnormality. Unmotivated, meaningless repetition of words and phrases.
Eclampsia	Hypertensive toxaemia affecting mother during last stage of pregnancy	Stillbirths common. Surviving infant may show severe brain damage and epileptic seizures. Can be severely retarded.
Encephalitis	Childhood viral infection leading to infection of brain substance	Acquired handicap. Damage to motor and intellectual functions wide range of subnormality.

Condition	Causes	Clinical features
Epilepsy *(Grand mal)*	Neurological malfunction (genetic or acquired), organic lesion	Often combined with subnormality. Continuous, massive bouts of fitting can produce organic damage. Characterized by sudden loss of consciousness accompanied by convulsions. May be preceded by sensory hallucinations. Characteristic EEG abnormality.
Galactosaemia	Single recessive gene. Congenital. Disorder of carbohydrate metabolism	Shortly after birth, vomiting and loss of appetite. Survivors are small and undernourished and may show mental handicap. Rare. Treatment by galactose-free diet until puberty.
Gargoylism I (Hurler's syndrome) II	Single recessive gene. Disorder of carbohydrate metabolism. Sex-linked recessive, affecting males	Mucopolysaceharide deposits in tissue cells of various organs. Physically grotesque appearance, enlarged head and forehead, dwarfism, protruding abdomen. Degree of retardation varies.
Gaucher's disease	Recessive gene, or simple dominant. Disorder of lipid metabolism	Enlargement of lymph-nodes, liver and spleen. Brain may be involved in acute onset and result in mental retardation. Uncommon.
Heller's disease (Dementia infantilis)	Metabolic disorder	Progressive atrophy of brain cells with deterioration of intellectual function. Dramatic decay within 9 months. Hyperactivity, stereotyped behaviour.
Homocystinura	Recessive genetic abnormality. Spontaneous genetic mutation. Disorder of amino acid metabolism	Physical abnormalities; fine hair, skeletal changes, and convulsions, often associated with mental handicap.
Huntington's chorea	Inherited, dominant gene	Half of offspring affected. Age of onset around 36, but can occur in childhood.˙ Progressive deterioration of function, usually intellectual first to break down.

Condition	Causes	Clinical features
Hydrocephalus	Developmental abnormality — excessive secretion CSF. Ventricular lesion. Meningitis. Spina bifida. (May be congenital, and may involve genetic factor)	Abnormal accumulation of cerebral spinal fluid (CSF) in ventricle and/or subarachnoid space. Symptoms include progressive enlargement of head, thinning of skull, atrophy of brain, convulsions and mental impairment. Condition may be arrested by early surgical intervention (e.g. Spitz-Holter valve).
Hypoglycaemia	Genetic. Mother — diabetes mellitus — eclampsia. Disorder of glucose metabolism	Premature babies and twins. Symptoms include reluctance to feed, convulsions, irritability. Treatment by diet.
Hypertelorism (Greig's syndrome)	Possible dominant gene and/or mutation. Cranial abnormality	Developmental abnormality of skull, physical deformity — eyes on side of face, hare lip, heart disease. May occur in association with other condition e.g. Down's syndrome. Severe cases usually associated with mental handicap.
Ichthyosis	Congenital, genetic (most frequently autosomal dominant)	Occurs in normal population. Sjorgren-Harsson syndrome — spasticity and mental handicap. Rud's syndrome — sexual infantilism, epilepsy, varying degrees of mental handicap.
Kernicterus	Blood toxins during antenatal period	Incompatible blood groups. Cyanosis. Without complete blood change — severe subnormality.
Klinefelter's syndrome	Sex chromosome abnormality (XXY)	Physical features — atrophied testicles and sterility, narrow shoulders, breasts may be feminine in appearance, long legs. Usually mild mental handicap, though often within normal range.
Laurence-Moon-Biedl syndrome	Possibly recessive gene	Characteristics — obesity, hypogenitalism, extra digits, eye defects, severe mental handicap. Close relatives may show signs. Rare.
Lead poisoning (Encephalopathy)	Ingestion/absorption	Morbid symptoms of CNS, including epileptiform convulsions, acute mania, delirium, coma. May lead to mental handicap. Treatment by chelating drugs after withdrawal from exposure.

Condition	Causes	Clinical features
Maple syrup urine disease	Congenital disorder of amino-acid metabolism	Urine has sweet smell resembling maple syrup. Blood contains abnormal amounts of valine, leucine, and isoleucine. Respiratory and feeding difficulties, stiffness of limbs. Rapid physical deterioration and death. Treatment by diet deficient in amino-acids.
Meningitis	Infection of meninges	Mental handicap may be a direct result of severe brain damage caused by meningitis, or indirectly from hydrocephalus occurring secondary to inflammation.
Microcephaly	Single recessive gene. Exposure to radiation	Inability of brain to develop normally. Head and brain much reduced in size. Spasticity and epilepsy are common. Variable mental handicap. May be a feature of other conditions.
Niemann-Pick disease	Recessive gene disorder of lipid metabolism	Characterized by physical and mental deterioration. Onset during infancy, often results in death before second year.
Patau's syndrome	Chromosome abnormality (Trisomy 13-15)	Gross malformation of the brain, severe mental retardation and early death.
Phenylketonuria	Autosomal recessive gene. Disorder of amino-acid metablolism	Absence of enzyme converting phenylalanine into tyrosine. Pigment deficiency, therefore patients usually fair. Sometimes have eczema, and show cyanosis of limbs. Epilepsy often occurs. Dietary treatment to avoid organic deterioration and severe subnormality.
Schilder's disease	Recessive gene	Progressive degeneration of nervous system associated with defective synthesis of myelin. Progressive mental impairment, ending in death.
Sturge-Weber's syndrome (naevoid amentia)	Causative factor unknown	Red or purple naevus on one side of face, occasionally involving same side of body. Naevus is of capillary-venous, angiomatous type. Menigeal angioma, epilepsy, contralateral hemiplegia. Treatment for epilepsy and sometimes surgical removal of naevus. Degree of mental handicap varies.
Triple X syndrome	Sex chromosome abnormality (XXX)	Female, showing no physical abnormalities. Variable mental handicap. Various psychotic disorders.

Condition	Causes	Clinical features
Tuberous sclerosis (epiloia)	Single dominant gene	Classic signs — mental retardation, epilepsy, adenoma sebaceum, though may be absent. Growths in brain and other organs may become malignant. Progressive mental deterioration with death often before maturity.
Turner's syndrome	Sex chromosome abnormality (OX)	Females with single X chromosome. Dwarfed, webbed neck, no ovaries. No sexual development at puberty. Mental retardation usually mild. Oestrogen replacement therapy.
XYY syndrome	Sex chromosome abnormality	Unusually tall, suggested tendency towards aggression and deviant behaviour. High incidence in security institutions. Sometimes reduction in intelligence.
Lesch-Nyan's syndrome	X-linked recessive chromosome condition	Characterized by spasticity and athetosis. Self-mutilation is common. Gout-like features. Hyperuicaemia.

†Bibliography: Dutton (1975); Hallas, Fraser, and Macgillivray (1974); Kirman and Bidwell (1975); Mackay (1976); Salmon (1978).

Appendix 2

Drug use in mental handicap

Drugs have a place only in the management of psychiatric disorders or physical conditions found in association with mental handicap, i.e. as an adjunct therapy, since, of course, mental handicap as such is not amenable to drug treatment and it is more appropriate to talk of management and training rather than drug treatment of this condition.

The prevalence of psychiatric disorders is greater in a mentally handicapped population than in the general population. For example take schizophrenia, a psychotic disorder which is found in about 1 per cent of the general population. In a mentally handicapped in-patient population the figure has been found to be around 2.5-3 per cent (Reid 1972; Heaton-Ward 1977). Neurotic illness has also a considerably higher prevalence amongst the mentally handicapped than in those of normal intelligence. After an accurate diagnosis has been made the appropriate drug therapy is instituted.

Most psychotropic drugs have as one of their side effects the action of sedating or slowing down motor activity, speech, and thought processes. There are one or two exceptions which are important in the field of mental handicap because these people can least of all afford the problems that accompany these unfortunate side effects. For instance, sodium valproate (trade name, 'Epilim') is used in anti-convulsant treatment and seems to be a useful drug in the management of several types of epileptic disorders. Lithium deserves a special mention as it is an extremely effective drug in the management of difficult, hostile, aggressive behaviour in sub-normal people — it controls without sedating. There are a number of drugs used in the management of depressive illnesses. These are known as the tricyclic group. For example, Imipramine (trade name 'Tofranil') is used to combat depression where motor retardation is a major effect, i.e. it has an alerting action. Another is amitriptyline (trade names, 'Lentizol', 'Tryptizol') which has a more sedative effect and would be used in treating agitated depression.

Finally when an accurate psychiatric diagnosis has been made, one would use the smallest dose of the appropriate drug necessary to control the symptoms, bearing in mind that the side-effects of psychotropic drugs are sometimes more troublesome and distressing than the condition for which it is prescribed. As Brian Kirman (1975) points out, there is much over-prescribing and the choice of drugs is not always logical. Monitoring of dosages needs to be part of routine practice in drug therapy with the mentally handicapped. With the exception of a few specific indications, the use of sedatives and tranquillizers for the mentally handicapped should only be employed as a temporary action until an alternative form of therapy can be adopted.

Appendix 3

Self assessment training questionnaire

Here are a number of questions surrounding situations you may find cropping up in your day-to-day work. Please tick the box you think provides the most appropriate answer and the way you would deal with the situation.

1. The emotional needs of handicapped children are:
    - (a) Completely different from other children ☐
    - (b) Do not exist ☐
    - (c) Like those of normal children ☐
    - (d) Less than those of other children ☐
2. A reward is given:
    - (a) When you think the child deserves it ☐
    - (b) Immediately after child shows desired behaviour ☐
    - (c) To keep a child quiet ☐
    - (d) To coax a child to give you desired behaviour ☐
3. When you are trying to stop a child having tantrums, the first thing to do is:
    - (a) Increase his medication ☐
    - (b) Make him stand in a corner ☐
    - (c) Observe and record his behaviour ☐
    - (d) Try to calm him down ☐
4. The most practical way of helping a child is to work with his behaviour. Which of the following are descriptions of behaviour?
    - (a) 'David is very aggressive' ☐
    - (b) 'David knows he is wrong' ☐
    - (c) 'David is clapping' ☐
    - (d) 'David's been bad today' ☐
5. Most behaviour is:
    - (a) Inherited ☐
    - (b) Due to growing up ☐
    - (c) Based on feelings ☐
    - (d) Learnt ☐

6. Once we have recorded and assessed behaviour:
   - (a) We have helped to train the child ☐
   - (b) We plan for appropriate action/therapy ☐
   - (c) We assess another child ☐
   - (d) We know more about the feelings of the mentally handicapped child ☐

7. A primary reward is:
   - (a) Sweets ☐
   - (b) Praise ☐
   - (c) Mini-bus outings ☐
   - (d) Shouting 'No' ☐

8. To find out whether a programme is working or not:
   - (a) You need a good memory ☐
   - (b) You need to make a snap decision ☐
   - (c) You need to have insight ☐
   - (d) You need to check your records of the child's behaviour ☐

9. You are trying to train a child. To date you have used gestural prompts without success. Your next step is to:
   - (a) Reward/reinforce the child ☐
   - (b) Go on to use physical prompts ☐
   - (c) Ignore it ☐
   - (d) Use sign language ☐

10. The children in your group are playing quietly. The thing to do is:
    - (a) Leave them alone ☐
    - (b) Turn on the television ☐
    - (c) Actively reward them for what they are doing ☐
    - (d) Tell them to stop being so quiet ☐

11. A secondary reward is:
    - (a) Ice cream ☐
    - (b) Fruit juice ☐
    - (c) Dancing ☐
    - (d) Medicine ☐

12. Reinforcement:
    - (a) Strengthens behaviour ☐
    - (b) Weakens the behaviour it follows ☐
    - (c) Strengthens the behaviour it follows ☐
    - (d) Weakens the behaviour it comes before ☐

13. Richard has temper tantrums because:
    - (a) He inherited a bad temper ☐
    - (b) He gets upset easily ☐
    - (c) His tantrums are reinforced ☐
    - (d) He has red hair ☐

14. Most people behave differently in different situations because:
    - (a) They are forced to ☐
    - (b) They like it ☐
    - (c) They have learnt to ☐
    - (d) They are all different from each other ☐

15. Building up a sequence of behaviour in therapy is called:
    (a) Tracking
    (b) Teaching
    (c) Shaping
    (d) Cajoling
16. Reducing the frequency of behaviour in therapy is called:
    (a) Short-cutting
    (b) Extinction
    (c) Reward removal
    (d) Successive approximation
17. Punishment:
    (a) Aims to make life unpleasant for people
    (b) Is concerned with methods to reduce behaviour
    (c) Is damaging to a person for the rest of their lives
    (d) Means getting someone to show that they are sorry
        for what they have done
18. Tick those of the following that are therapy techniques:
    (a) Calming down
    (b) Reward presentation
    (c) Backward chaining
    (d) Penalty removal
    (e) Modelling
    (f) Therapy planning
    (g) Fading out
19. A schedule of continuous positive reinforcement means:
    (a) Using penalties immediately after a fixed period of time
        to increase a specific behaviour
    (b) Employing rewards immediately after each time a specific
        behaviour occurs to achieve reinforcement
    (c) Whenever you see someone you are working with you say,
        'that's good' or similar statements
    (d) Continuously changing the time you reward someone
20. A schedule of continuous negative reinforcement means:
    (a) Punishing someone so they will 'behave themselves' in the
        future
    (b) Constantly taking things the person likes away from them
    (c) Criticizing someone whenever you get the chance
    (d) Immediately removing penalties when appropriate
        behaviour occurs
21. Interval reinforcement is practised by:
    (a) Waiting until you feel it's about time you tried to reinforce
        an individual's behaviour
    (b) Waiting a pre-selected period of time, at the end of which
        rewards are presented or penalties removed to achieve
        reinforcement
    (c) Counting up to ten then rewarding the person to achieve
        reinforcement
    (d) Sending the person into a corner for five minutes

22. Ratio reinforcement is practised by:
    (a) Finding out how much a person likes a reward before you reinforce them ☐
    (b) Using six or seven rewards to reinforce someone every time a target behaviour occurs ☐
    (c) Employing more primary rewards than secondary rewards to achieve reinforcement ☐
    (d) Applying rewards or removing penalties immediately after a predetermined number of times a behaviour occurs ☐
23. Plotting graphs:
    (a) Are a waste of valuable time ☐
    (b) Don't tell us anything we don't know already ☐
    (c) Provide accurate information about a person's behaviour before, during, and after therapy ☐
    (d) Help us to decide which therapy techniques to use ☐
24. Continuous assessment should:
    (a) Aim to tell us everything about a person ☐
    (b) Aim to apply a system of constant checks which provides information about the different stages of the therapeutic management model ☐
    (c) Establish a method of working which permits an ever changing set of therapy targets to be used in therapy ☐
25. The therapeutic management model permits the therapist to evaluate (tick any answers you think are appropriate):
    (a) Assessment and observation ☐
    (b) Therapy formulations ☐
    (c) Therapeutic practice ☐
    (d) Continuous assessment ☐
    (e) None of the items in this section ☐
    (f) All of the items in this section ☐

Now that you have completed the Self Assessment Training Questionnaire discuss your results with your colleagues and tutors. Clarify any misunderstandings and repeat completion of a corrected questionnaire where necessary. Conclude this exercise by showing how the ideas expressed in the questionnaire might be seen and used in nursing practice.

References and further reading

References marked with an asterisk are recommended further reading.

BAILEY, R. and PATERSON, R. (1977). When care alone is not enough. *Apex* **5**, 4-7.

*BANDURA, A. (1969). *Principles of behavior modification.* Holt, Rinehart, & Winston, New York.

*BARNARD, K. E. and ERIKSON, M. L. (1976). *Teaching children with developmental problems: a family care approach.* C. V. Mosby, St. Loius.

*CLARKE, A. M. and CLARKE, A. D. B. (1974). *Mental deficiency: the changing outlook.* Methuen, London.

*COMLEY, J. (1975). *Behaviour modification with the retarded child.* Heinemann Medical Books, London.

*DUTTON, G. (1975). *Mental handicap.* Butterworths, London.

*ERIKSON, E. H. (1973). *Childhood and society.* Penguin, Harmondsworth.

*GARDNER, W. I. (1972). *Behaviour modification in mental retardation: the education and rehabilitation of the mentally retarded adolescent and adult.* University of London Press.

*GUNZBURG, H. C. (1973). *Social competence and mental handicap.* Ballière Tindall, London.

*HALLAS, C. H., FRASER, W. I., and MACGILLIVRAY, R. C. (1974). *The care and training of the mentally handicapped* (5th edn). John Wright, Bristol.

HEATON-WARD, A. (1977). *Psychosis in mental handicap.* The Tenth Blance Marsh Lecture. *Br. J. Psychiat.* **130**, 525-33.

HMSO (1971). *Better services for the mentally handicapped.* Cmnd 4683. Her Majesty's Stationery Office, London.

*ILLINGWORTH, R. S. (1974). *The development of the infant and young child: normal and abnormal.* Churchill Livingstone, Edinburgh.

Institute of Mental Subnormality (1977). *Ethical implications for behavioral modification.* Institute of Mental Subnormality, Kidderminster.

*JEFFREE, D. M., McKONKEY, R. and HEWSON, S. (1978). *Teaching the handicapped child.* Human Horizon Series. Souvenir Press, London.

*KIRMAN, P. (1975). *Mental handicap. A brief guide.* Crosby Lockwood Staples, London.

—— (1975). Drug therapy in mental handicap. *Br. J. Psychiat.* **127**, 545-9.

—— and BICKNELL, J. (1975). *Mental handicap.* Churchill Livingstone, Edinburgh.

*KIERNAN, C., JORDAN, R., and SAUNDRES, C. (1978). *Starting off. Establishing play and communication in the handicapped child.* Human Horizon Series. Souvenir Press, London.

LUNZER, E. A. (1970). *On children thinking.* Inaugural lecture, Department of Education, University of Nottingham. National Foundation for Educational Research, Slough.

MACKAY, R. I. (1976). *Mental handicap in child health practice.* Butterworth, London.

*PEINE, H. A. and HOWARTH, R. (1976). *Children and parents. Everyday problems of behaviour.* Penguin, Harmondsworth.

*PERKINS, E. A. TAYLOR, P. D., and CAPIE, A. C. M. (1978). *Helping the retarded.* British Institute of Mental Handicap Publications, Kidderminster.

REID, A. H. (1972). Psychoses in adult mental defectives: I Manic depressive psychosis. *Br. J. Psychiat.* **120,** 205-12.

SALMON, M.A. (1978). *Developmental defects and syndromes.* H.M. & M. Publishers, Aylesbury.

*SCHAEFER, C. E. and MILLMAN, J. L. (1977). *Therapies for children.* Jossey-Bass, San Francisco.

*SHAKESPEARE, R. (1975). *Essential psychology: the psychology of handicap.* Associated Book Publishers, London.

*STEPHENS, T. M. (1970). *Directive teaching of children with learning and behavioral handicaps.* Charles Merril, Ohio.

*STERN, R. (1973). *Behavioural techniques. A therapist's manual.* Academic Press, New York.

*STEVENS, M. (1978a). *Observe — then teach. An observational approach to teaching mentally handicapped children.* Arnold, London.

*—— (1978b). *The educational and social needs of children with severe handicap.* Arnold, London.

TROWER, P., BRYANT, B., and ARGYLE, M. (1978). *Social skills and mental health.* Methuen, London.

WALKER, M. (1980). *The Makaton vocabulary.* The Makaton vocabulary Development Project, London.

*WATSON, L. S. (1972). *How to use behavior modification with mentally retarded and autistic children. Programmes for administrators, teachers, parents, and nurses.* Behaviour Modification Technology Inc., Illinois.

*WHELAN, E. and SPEAKE, B. (1979). *Learning to cope.* Human Horizon series. Souvenir Press, London.

ZAAGWILL, O. L. (ed.) (1980). *Behaviour modification.* Report of a joint working party. HMSO, London.

Addresses

American Association on Mental Deficiency	5201-5101 Wisconsin Avenue, NW Washington DC 20016, USA.
Adaptive Behaviour Scale	By Kazuo Nihra, Ph.D. New Psychiatric Institute, University of California, 7660 Westwood Place, Los Angeles, CA 90024, USA.
The Developmental Checklist	By E. A. Perkins, P. D. Taylor, and A. C. M. Copie. Available from The British Institute of Mental Handicap [formerly Institute of Mental Subnormality], Wolverhampton Road, Kidderminster, Worcs. DY10 3PP.
Progress Assessment Chart (P-A-C)	By Dr H. C. Gunzburg.

UK
NSMHC — Books, 17 Pembridge Hall, 17 Pembridge Square, London W2 4EP. Tel: 01-229 8941.

Australia
Australian Council for Educational Research, Frederick Street, Hawthorn E2, Victoria 3122. Tel: 811271.

Canada
ASH/Deerhome, P-A-C Dept., PO Box 5002 — Red Deer, Alberta T4N 5H1. Tel: 403/347-4455.

Holland
Swets and Zeitlinger, Heereweg 3476, 2160 AH Lisse, Holland.

New Zealand
New Zealand Council for Educational Research, Box 3237, Wellington, NZ.

USA
Aux Chandelles, P-A-C Dept., PO Box 398 — Bristol Indiana 46507. Tel: (219) 848-7451.

Parent Involvement Project developmental charts (PIP)	By Dorothy M. Jeffree and Roy McConkey. Hester Adrian Research Centre, University of Manchester. Available from Hodder and Stoughton (Educational), Dunton Green, Sevenoaks, Kent TN13 2YD.
Raeden Assessment Scales	The Raeden Centre, Midstocket Road, Aberdeen AB2 4PE.

Index